Selected Topics on Infant Feeding

Edited by Isam Jaber AL-Zwaini and Haider Hadi AL-Musawi

Published in London, United Kingdom

Selected Topics on Infant Feeding
http://dx.doi.org/10.5772/intechopen.98106
Edited by Isam Jaber AL-Zwaini and Haider Hadi AL-Musawi

Contributors
Margarita Manosalvas, Ka-Huen Yip, Mei-Kuen Chow, Yuk-Chiu Yip, Wai-King Tsui, Inna Vladimirovna Simakova, Ekaterina Yurievna Volf, Andrey Anatolyevich Terentyev, Aleksandr Sergeevich Fedonnikov, Nina Viktorovna Bolotova, Gloria Vladimirovna Guzeeva, Viktor Veniaminovich Zakrevsky, Enos Mirembe Masereka, Clement Munguiko, Alex Tumusiime, Linda Grace Alanyo, Sunil Jain, Arvind Singh Kushwaha, Vishal Marwaha

First published in London, United Kingdom, 2022 by IntechOpen
IntechOpen is the global imprint of INTECHOPEN LIMITED, registered in England and Wales, registration number: 11086078, 5 Princes Gate Court, London, SW7 2QJ, United Kingdom

British Library Cataloguing-in-Publication Data
A catalogue record for this book is available from the British Library

Additional hard and PDF copies can be obtained from orders@intechopen.com

Selected Topics on Infant Feeding
Edited by Isam Jaber AL-Zwaini and Haider Hadi AL-Musawi
p. cm.
Print ISBN 978-1-80355-789-2
Online ISBN 978-1-80355-790-8
eBook (PDF) ISBN 978-1-80355-791-5

Meet the editors

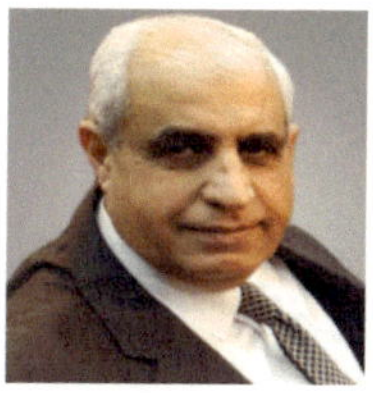

Prof. Isam Jaber AL-Zwaini graduated from AL-Mustansiryia College of Medicine, Iraq, in 1987, after which he worked as a house officer in different hospitals in Baghdad for fifteen months followed by military service for three years. He began his pediatrics study in 1991 and obtained a fellowship from the Iraqi Commission for Medical Specializations in 1996. He was a lecturer in the Department of Pediatrics, AL-Anbar College of Medicine, Iraq, from 1996 to 2001, after which he was promoted to assistant professor. In 2005, he began working in the Department of Pediatrics, Al-Kindy College of Medicine, University of Baghdad, Iraq. He became a professor there in 2008. Prof. AL-Zwaini was head of the Department of Pediatrics at both AL-Anbar and AL-Kindy Medical Colleges for many years. He is a member of the Royal College of Pediatrics and Child Health, UK. He has published more than thirty scientific papers in different pediatric fields and has a special interest in pediatric hematology, neurology, and nutrition.

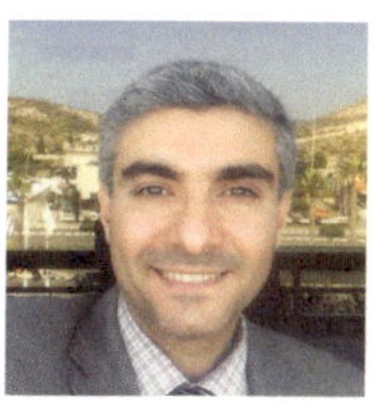

Dr. Hayder Hadi AL-Musawi is a member of the Pediatrics Department, Al-Kindy College of Medicine, University of Baghdad, Iraq. He is a consultant pediatrician practicing at Al-Elwiya Pediatric Teaching Hospital, Baghdad. He has published more than twenty-five papers in national and international scientific journals. He is a Scopus-certified scientific reviewer and a member of many associations worldwide including the British Association for Child Health (BACCH) and the British Special Interest Group.

Contents

Preface

The growth and development of infants during the first two years of life are greatly influenced by nutrition. Meeting basic nutritional requirements is vital for proper and optimal growth and development, both physically and mentally. Infant feeding practice has greatly changed since the beginning of the last century. Many factors have influenced the rate of breastfeeding and the proper timing of complementary feed introduction. Poverty, world wars, the influx of women in the workforce, and the development of commercial infant formula are among these factors. Feeding during the first 1000 days of life is crucial for the growth and development of an individual and their long-term health outcomes. On many occasions, major nutritional problems such as obesity and undernutrition have been linked to nutrition during infancy. These problems not only affect the individual but also impact the future of developing countries. In four sections containing five chapters, this book discusses selected topics on infant feeding.

Chapter 1 by Jain et al. discusses the need for universal health care for all infants. The authors state that exclusively breastfeeding for the first six months, then for two or more years with proper weaning, is desirable. As such, the authors propose the 'ABC mothers' plan.

In Chapter 2, Masereka et al. discuss infant and young child feeding in developing countries. Infant feeding challenges continue to manifest in developed and developing countries. Worldwide, more than 80% of babies are breastfed in the first few weeks of birth. However, about 37%, 25%, and less than 1% are exclusively breastfed at 6 months of age in Africa, the United States, and the United Kingdom, respectively. These statistics are far below the World Health Organization targets of 50% by 2025 and 70% by 2030. Complementary feeding practices are varied as well due to non-adherence to infant and young child feeding guidelines among parents.

Chapter 3 by Manosalvas discusses the causes of policy failure to reduce chronic childhood undernutrition in Ecuador during a period of economic growth. The overall reduction of undernutrition from 1999 to the time of writing this chapter is 0.83 percent per year. Surprisingly, the period of highest GDP between 2006 and 2014, in which Ecuador exhibited economic growth of more than 4% of GDP per year on average, showed a lesser reduction in childhood malnutrition of only 0.2 percent per year. The author uses a mixed research strategy to explain this paradox.

Chapter 4 by Ka-Huen et al. discusses the issue of breastfeeding during the COVID-19 pandemic in Hong Kong. As new mothers are understandably concerned about COVID-19 and its high rate of infection, they are often unsure if they should breastfeed their infants. In general, hospitals do not allow direct breastfeeding by mothers with an active infection of SARS-CoV-2. Some neonatal units in Hong Kong maintain safe practices by isolating infants and mothers for at least 7 to 14 days, even if the infant remains SARS-CoV-2 negative. During isolation, mothers encourage the expression of milk to maintain milk duct patency and to prepare for lactation when they and their infants are discharged.

Finally, Chapter 5 by Volf et al. presents the authors' original research on fat component safety and pre-clinical evaluation of the physiological effect of infant-adapted dry milk mixtures. The fat component is one of the key components of an infant's diet. Its important aspects are biological effectiveness and safety changes during processing, storage, transportation, and subsequent storage after opening the package. Consumption of oxidized fats leads to pathological changes in the organism.

We would like to thank all the contributing authors for their excellent chapters and for their patience and cooperation. Furthermore, I would like to express my gratitude and sincere appreciation to the staff at IntechOpen, especially Author Service Manager Iva Ribic for her assistance throughout the publication process.

Isam Jaber AL-Zwaini
Professor,
Department of Pediatrics,
AL-Kindy College of Medicine,
University of Baghdad,
Baghdad, Iraq

Haider Hadi AL-Musawi
Assistant Professor,
Department of Pediatrics,
AL-Kindy College of Medicine,
University of Baghdad,
Baghdad, Iraq

Section 1

Successful Breast Feeding; Implementation Strategies

Chapter 1

'Complete Coverage & Covering Completely' for Breastfeeding with Able, Bold, & Confident Mothers, for Sustainable Development, & Medical Education Excellence

Sunil Jain, Arvind Singh Kushwaha and Vishal Marwaha

Abstract

Complete coverage of all infants, everywhere with wonderful evidence, and covering completely with first six months of exclusive breastfeeding and thereafter proper weaning while continuing breastfeeding up to 2 years of age or beyond is desirable. Reaching all rightly and robustly is required. All this will contribute greatly towards the growth & development of infants and grandly towards the Sustainable Development Goals. We propose the "ABC mothers" plan. Progress for required practices for results possible with making mothers—"Able for practices advantageous, bold with pertinent awareness, and confident with propitious attitude". Strong efforts on sound footing are necessary for health of all our infants and happiness all around with sustainable development. Scientific infant feeding will contribute to advance the attainment of this. Medical education teaching best beneficial practices is for excellence. One promoting breastfeeding is the best. The US Surgeon General's Implementation Strategies elaborate "Education content", "Enabling competency", & "Education continuing". Competency-based curriculum for Indian Medical Graduates includes "to promote and support optimal breast feeding". Need for inclusion in teaching curriculum across US, UK, & internationally has been documented. Given all the evidence for breastfeeding benefits, it should be a consistent essential component of training in all medical schools worldwide.

Keywords: complementary feeding, weaning, maternity leave, preterm, surrogacy, knowledge, skills, regulations, teaching, competency

1. Introduction

Infants and young children are the beginning of the ambitions of life. All health plans for them should be ambitious, vigorous, & vivacious. Breastfeeding is an excellent start for children. All babies should be breastfed, with the motto "cover all & cover completely", motivating all concerned, & with the motive of achieving excellence, with complete coverage. Early initiation of breastfeeding, exclusive breastfeeding for first six months, followed by timely, adequate, safe, and appropriate complementary feeding, while continuing breastfeeding up to 2 years of age or beyond is recommended. Starting within the first hour of birth, longer-duration breastfeeding is associated with protection against childhood infections, increases in intelligence & reductions in the prevalence of overweight and diabetes [1]. Breastfeeding is associated with improved performance in intelligence tests 30 years later and might have an important effect in real life, by increasing educational attainment and income in adulthood [2]. Innovations are needed to accelerate progress for our children's health & there is a need to involve everyone. For their future and the future of our world [3]. Best breastfeeding policies & practices will advance the attainment of the Sustainable Development Goals (SDGs). Medical education excellence is teaching best beneficial practices, which prominently includes breastfeeding.

2. Able, bold, & confident mothers

The success of breastfeeding initiation and continuation depends on multiple factors, such as education about breastfeeding, preparation for breastfeeding, hospital breastfeeding practices and policies, routine and timely follow-up care, and family and societal support. Maternal breastfeeding self-efficacy is a significant predictor of breastfeeding duration and level [4]. Mothers may need help to adopt better practices, or to overcome difficulties with their own health, nutrition, or family planning [5]. Mothers are at the center stage for breast & complementary feeding. Hence, we propose the ABC plan of breast and complementary feeding—Able, Bolder, and Confident mothers

2.1 Able

It is important to make all mothers able to breastfeed, with all the correct knowledge, positive attitude, and reinforced support for breast and complementary feeding. This should be done with all the promptness with which the CPR (Cardio-Pulmonary Resuscitation) is done, as this is the factor of core importance for preventing all morbidities and mortalities. This is the beginning of life and should be a healthy beginning.

To be ably breastfeed, mothers' own health is important. Various aspects to be taken care of include nutritional status and food intake, any illness she may have, maternal medications, birth spacing, and family planning. Emotional & social support to the mothers is important.

The energy cost of breastfeeding should be catered for. A mother's intake should be increased by around 10% in women not physically active. The increase should be 20% or more in moderately or very active women. Poor diet, quantitatively or qualitatively affects mothers' energy and ability to breastfeed or to feed and care for their infant or child. A lactating mother needs around 500 kilocalories (roughly equivalent to one extra meal) each day for making 750 ml of breast milk. The required nutrients are supplied from body stores partly, laid down during pregnancy. The rest need to be supplied as an increased intake [6]. All this is ensured by greater amount and variety of foods. Pregnant and lactating women can eat any foods normally included in the local diet.

The Baby-Friendly Hospital Initiative (BFHI) comprehensively enables mothers to breastfeed, as systematic ten steps. Evidence exists for the effectiveness of individual steps, but even more so for full implementation of all steps together [7–9]. The ten steps to successful breastfeeding of BFHI are:

1. a. Compliance: full to International Code of Marketing of Breast-milk Substitutes and relevant World Health Assembly resolutions.

   b. Written policy: on infant feeding routinely communicated to staff and parents.

   c. Ongoing monitoring and data-management systems: are in place.

2. Trained staff: having sufficient knowledge, competence, and skills to support breastfeeding.

3. Counselling: for importance and management of breastfeeding with pregnant women and their families.

4. Initiation: immediate and uninterrupted skin-to-skin contact is facilitated. Mothers are supported for initiation of breastfeeding as soon as possible after birth.

5. Support: for mothers to maintain breastfeeding and manage common difficulties.

6. Exclusive guidance: for not to provide breastfed newborns any food or fluids other than breast milk, unless medically indicated.

7. Rooming-in: enable mothers and their infants to remain together 24 hours a day.

8. Infant cues: teach mothers to recognize and respond to their infants' cues for feeding.

9. Counselling additional: on the use and risks of feeding bottles, teats & pacifiers.

10. Care ongoing: coordination of discharge so that parents and their infants have timely access to ongoing support [10].

Baby-friendly and biological nurturing approach has been shown to be highly effective [11]. Biological nurturing is a neurobehavioral approach to breastfeeding support. It encourages women to breastfeed in a relaxed, laidback position. This approach is advantageous with reduction in breast problems (e.g., sore nipples), making good latch easier and thus facilitating the initiation of exclusive breastfeeding [12].

Social support is required and results in success contributing to making mothers able to breastfeed. These should include emotional, tangible, and educational components. Providers of these should include both informal social network members (male partner, mother, family/friends) and professional network members (health care professionals, lactation consultants). Also, negative social support may decrease breastfeeding [13].

Breastfeeding is an intimate process that requires psychosocial adjustment as well as technical skills. During these adjustments, psychological support will contribute to success [14].

Couples need to be advised to wait at least 24 months after a live birth and 6 months after a miscarriage before attempting the next pregnancy [15]. This ensures mothers' health, good birth weight, & ability to breast & complementary feed in the desired way.

Also, correct advice is required if mother becomes pregnant while breastfeeding. This mostly occurs when the breastfeeding infant is older than 6 months. After this age dependency on mother for nutritional needs is not total as weaning has started. Breastfeeding during pregnancy is thought to pose no increased risk to the pregnancy [16].

Mothers can face challenges in breastfeeding. Conquering the challenges is important for making them able to breastfeed. The American College of Obstetricians & Gynecologists (ACOG) has comprehensively made detailed recommendations and conclusions regarding breastfeeding challenges [17]. Obstetrician–gynecologists and other obstetric care professionals are uniquely positioned to support women in these situations [17].

Able mothers practicing correct breast & complementary feeding will help in achieving nutrition and health goals.

2.2 Bold

Making women bold is the way forward. Correct knowledge will make mothers bold & bold mothers will not deviate from correct practices. Antenatal counseling sessions giving knowledge & skills of scientific practices will make them ready for the very best implementation. Large-scale interventions focusing on educating mothers about breastfeeding have the potential to increase breastfeeding prevalence. A systematic review on breastfeeding interventions has concluded that combined individual and group counseling appeared to be superior to individual or group counseling alone [18]. This will ensure breastfeeding with desired confidence.

The logic of correct knowledge-making mothers bold is illustrated by following examples. The WHO Integrated Management of Neonatal and Childhood Illness (IMNCI) “feeding recommendations during sickness and health” are:

i. Up to 6 months of Age: Breastfeed as often as the child wants, day and night, at least 8 times in 24 hours.

ii. 6 months up to 24 months: Breastfeed as often as the child wants.

Remember: Continue breastfeeding if the child is sick

If breastfeeding, exclusive and continued, in sickness is beneficial then mothers will definitely be bold for breastfeeding. IMNCI implementation in Real Life Situation is strongly recommended [19].

Another excellent example is hot conditions & deserts. It was generally, but wrongly, agreed that infants in a hot and dry climate need extra water. This assumption was based more on caution than on knowledge. An important study showed that breastfed infants in a hot and humid climate were found to do well without supplementary water [20]. Current recommendation is, breastfed infants do not require additional water. Correct knowledge will definitely empower mothers with boldness.

Working mother issues need to be addressed. ACOG recommends providing anticipatory guidance about how to continue breastfeeding after returning to work [17]. The

Maternity Benefit Act 1961 (amended up to 2017) has provided for "Nursing breaks"—"*Every woman delivered of a child who returns to duty after such delivery shall, in addition to the interval for rest allowed to her, be allowed in the course of her daily work two breaks of the prescribed duration for nursing the child until the child attains the age of fifteen months*" [21].

Breastfeeding in public, when required, needs to be taken care of. Women should feel at home in the world, and we should ensure this. This will also make their babies feel at home in the world. Mother work in public should be free, safe, & as full citizens without harassment or surveillance. Bold mothers are a prerequisite for all this.

Newspaper articles report & reflect current trends. A newspaper in India has recently, in an article titled "Bold & Breastfeeding", importantly reported "More and more Indian moms are confidently nursing in public and proudly sharing pictures online too" [22]. This is the right direction meeting the requirement to feed the baby when the baby wants and not disrupting mothers' life or freedom. In today's world Digital Communication aids reaching all and should contribute to popularizing right practices.

2.3 Confident

We need to infuse confidence into mothers that proper breast and complementary feeding will lead to healthier babies with bright futures. These practices rank among the most effective interventions to improve child health. The WHO systematic review of long-term effects of breastfeeding has concluded that there is strong evidence of a causal effect of breastfeeding on IQ [23]. All this positive evidence will infuse confidence for a propitious attitude and actions.

Confidence in the ability to breastfeed has been shown to be the most important predictor of full first six months of exclusive breastfeeding [24]

An increase in mothers' confidence in themselves, in breastfeeding, and in their infants' growth and development is simple & requires supporting mothers to respond in a variety of ways to behavioral cues for feeding, comfort, or closeness. This enables them to build caring, nurturing relationships with their infants. Ways to respond to infant cues include breastfeeding, skin-to-skin contact, cuddling, carrying, talking, singing, and so forth [25].

Alive & Thrive initiative addressed the multiple influences that can affect a mother's confidence and ability to optimally breastfeed [26]. The interventions included provision of training, supportive supervision, job aids, & communications materials to both health workers working at the primary care level (local health centers) and the volunteer community health worker cadre [27]. Health education reinforcement for healthy practices is the key and gives mothers necessary confidence.

Media plays an important role in our lives, and definitely should play a positive role to raise community awareness about the benefits of breastfeeding for both the mother and her baby. All this will make mothers confident about breastfeeding.

Social media breastfeeding support groups (SMBSGs) have been found to be useful. These have been found to improve women's confidence, knowledge, and attitudes and, therefore, increase the potential for exclusive breastfeeding to 6 months [28].

3. Special situations

Covering all is important and special situations demand specific considerations.

3.1 Preterm babies feeding

Premature infants receive profound benefits from breastfeeding [29]. Maternal breast milk should be the preferred enteral feeding for premature infants, although its nutritional adequacy may be limited for several reasons [30]. Preterm mothers' milk has greater protein content than that of mothers delivering at term, however, it is insufficient in meeting the needs of smaller and more immature preterm infants [31]. Human milk fortifier should be added once the premature infant is tolerating tube feeding, and its use should be continued until the infant has achieved all oral feedings, a weight of 1800 g, or is near to discharge from the hospital. Similarly, Very Low Birth Weight (VLBW) infants should receive a human milk fortifier. This meets their nutritional needs and prevents clinical deficiency diseases and growth failure.

3.2 Breastfeeding without birthing

Breastfeeding is all advantageous, and should also be done after surrogacy and adoption. There is a growing awareness that it is possible for women to breastfeed in these situations. Health care professionals should support these mothers. Breastfeeding can play a significant role in facilitating the development of the child-mother relationship in cases of adoption and surrogacy [32, 33]. This is besides all the physiological benefits.

Induction of lactation in the biological mother after gestational surrogacy and in cases of adoption is required. A combination of pharmacological and nonpharmacological methods is often used for the induction of lactation [34]. Medications to help induce lactation are useful. ACOG recommends that galactagogues may be helpful if a woman would like to produce milk for an adopted infant [17]. Various protocols for inducing lactation and maximizing milk production are there [35, 36].

4. Complementary feeding

The general principles of complementary feeding are:

i. Start: at six months

ii. Responsive feeding: needs to be practiced, applying the principles of psychosocial care

iii. Hygiene: good along with proper food handling

iv. Quantity: start with small amounts of food and increase the quantity as the child gets older, while maintaining frequent breastfeeding

v. Food type: food consistency to be gradually increased and variety added as the infant grows older, adapting to the infant's requirements and abilities. Introduce one food at a time

vi. Frequency: increase the number of times that the child is fed complementary foods as the child gets older

vii. Variety: feed a variety of nutrient-rich foods, ensuring that all nutrient needs are met.

viii. Source: locally available & home food recommended

ix. Energy density: should be more than that of breast milk

x. Technique: encourage cup and avoid bottle

xi. Illness & recovery: increase fluid intake during illness, including more frequent breastfeeding, and encourage the child to eat soft, favorite foods. After illness, give food more often than usual and encourage the child to eat more.

xii. Breastfeeding simultaneous: continue breastfeeding until 2 years of age or beyond.

Newborn babies have a right to survive and grow into childhood, and to experience life to their full potential [37]. With "ABC plan" mothers will be able to better and comprehensively contribute towards this. Proper nutrition is the first prerequisite for attaining full potential.

Overall, our ABC plan is summarized as:

'Able, bold, & confident mothers, for

All advantageous, best beneficial, bolstering comprehensive care'

5. Sustainable development goals with breast & complementary feeding

The SDGs are a collection of 17 interlinked global goals as a plan of action for people, planet, and prosperity. These are people-centered, universal, and transformative [38].

Breastfeeding-achieving the new normal is based on consolidation of evidence for breastfeeding's benefits in recent years, in particular, the economic gains to be reaped [39]. All advantages are contributory towards SDGs.

SDGs, adopted by the world leaders are expected to follow on from the Millennium Development Goals (MDGs). We need to accelerate our progress [3]. Breastfeeding and complementary feeding (BFCF) are important & the impact for attaining SDGs & all the MDGs is as follows:

- 'Eradicate extreme poverty and hunger' (SDG 1 & 2 / MDG 1)

Adequate and scientifically correct BFCF has tremendous potential for achieving progress in food and nutrition security in childhood, completely and comprehensibly. The savings from expenditure on other milk & its substitutes also contributes to "No poverty". High returns on health investments can aid to eliminate poverty. Protection, promotion, and support for breastfeeding results in savings totaling US$302 billion annually [40], i.e. nearly 0.5 percent of the world gross national industry.

Breastfeeding is a natural and economical way of feeding. It does not burden household budgets. Savings will contribute to feeding other household members resulting in no hunger and ultimately eradication of poverty.

- 'Good health & well-being' (SDG 3)

Optimal breastfeeding & complementary feeding ensures this not only for the present but also for the future. Breastfeeding confers short-term and long-term benefits for both child and mother, including helping to protect children against a variety of acute and chronic disorders. The benefits of breastfeeding are confirmed in fewer infections, increased intelligence, probable protection against overweight and diabetes, and cancer prevention for mothers [23, 39]. The short-term as well as long-term, disadvantages of not breastfeeding are important [23, 41].

- 'Quality education' (SDG 4) / 'Achieve universal primary education' (MDG 2)

Free from disease means fit to attend school on all days. The benefits of breastfeeding on good health & in preventing childhood morbidities are well proven.

Breastfeeding and quality complementary foods significantly contribute to cognitive development, support appropriate neurological development and enhance later school performance. Adequately BFCF will boost universal primary education, aptly and appropriately. All this will enormously contribute to global learning targets.

- "Gender equality" (SDG 5) / "Promote gender equality and empower women" (MDG 3)

Women should receive equality at all levels of society. Women's reproductive rights and productive roles require adequate support. Providing them with accurate information about BFCF will empower them, and provision of breastfeeding-friendly workplaces will make them practice it.

A study on breastfeeding has shown that interventions such as maternity leave, workplace support, and employment status of mothers led to a 30 percent increase in breastfeeding rates [42]. We all need to get the cycle going for best feeding practices for best goals accomplishments.

- "Reduce child mortality" (MDG 4)

For this, the importance of adequate BFCF practices is supported by a large body of scientific evidence. Breastfeeding provides protection against childhood infections along with other advantages. Early start and longer duration of breastfeeding as recommended are the most useful. Research has shown that scaling up breastfeeding up to near-universal levels will result in saving the lives of 823,000 children under age 5 in 75 low- and middle-income countries [1]. All this justifies implementation of breastfeeding recommendations with full devotion and diligently.

- 'Improve maternal health' (MDG 5)

Breastfeeding has a positive impact on the health of mothers. For nursing women, breastfeeding protects against breast cancer and improves birth spacing [1]. The more the mothers breastfeed, the greater are the benefits. These advantages of breastfeeding should be widely told simply and scientifically.

- "Combat HIV/AIDS, malaria and other diseases" (MDG 6)

The protective effects of breastfeeding against infections are well known. For HIV/AIDS, there is now enough evidence to recommend ARVs during breastfeeding. Research shows that HIV-positive mothers who receive effective ARV treatment can have a close to zero transmission rate of HIV to their babies during pregnancy, birth, and breastfeeding. Thus, breastfeeding will help reduce morbidity and mortality from infections dramatically and drastically.

- "Ensure access to affordable, reliable, sustainable, and modern energy for all" (SDG 7) / "Ensure environmental sustainability" (MDG 7)

The manufacture of breast milk substitute products and their packaging is a wasteful activity, which pollutes and damages the environment. The bottles not only degrade the health of the babies but are also non-biodegradable. Our recommended optimum BFCF will lead to environmental protection and preservation.

- "Decent work & economic growth" (SDG 8) & "Reduced inequalities" (SDG 10)

Breastfeeding is associated with adding US$302 billion annually in additional income to the world economy [40], in the healthiest way. All babies breastfed & given complementary feeding will definitely result in reduced inequalities.

- "Responsible consumption & production" (SDG 12)

Breastmilk does not require industry for the production and is created and consumed with a minimal ecological footprint. It is the healthiest consumption. Home-based locally available complementary feeds are again responsible for consumption & production.

- "Global partnerships for the goals" (SDG 17) / "Develop a global partnership for development" (MDG 8)

The promotion for optimum BFCF requires multi-sectoral collaboration. WHO, UNICEF, various government & non-government organizations cooperating for Infant feeding. This provides an opportunity for building on the existent international partnerships for support of development. A healthy start to life for all babies of the world is the best possible development which we should aim, support, and sustain.

All this is best summarized as:

> *'Scientific, energetic, & strong efforts for sustainable excellence,*
>
> *Breastfeeding is best and fruitful'*

6. Medical education: Methodical excellence

Excellent medical education is one that teaches best beneficial practices. BFCF is of importance for all our infants for lifelong benefits. Promoting correct practices is an imperative duty & important obligation. Advanced methodical learning and optimized learning lead to better-trained doctors [43].

The US Surgeon General in its *Call to Action to Support Breastfeeding* (2011) remarked [44]:

> *"Inadequate education and training of clinicians has been identified as a major barrier to breastfeeding, and*
> *education on breastfeeding is not a core element of most medical school or residency programs or of programs in nursing education."*

'*The US Surgeon General's Call to Action to Support Breastfeeding*' describes in detail the Implementation Strategies:

i. Education content: Improvements in the breastfeeding content in undergraduate and graduate education and ongoing training for health professionals. Quality content recommended.

ii. Enabling competency: Incorporation of competency in lactation care as minimum requirements for health professional credentialing, licensing, and certification processes.

iii. Education continuing: Increase opportunities for continuing education on the management of lactation to ensure the maintenance of minimum competencies and skills [44].

The Medical Council of India (now National Medical Commission of India) has effective outcome-based strategies. The MCI Competency-based Undergraduate curriculum for the Indian Medical Graduate [45] requires the following competency:

> *'To promote and support optimal Breastfeeding for Infants'*

This simple straightforward statement is all favorable, for all the life, for all the liveliness throughout life, & is the amongst the foremost best duty doctors can do.

The General Medical Council (GMC), UK, in its 'Outcomes for Medical Graduates' mentions [46]:

> *"Newly qualified doctors must be able to apply biomedical scientific principles, methods, and knowledge to medical practice and integrate these into patient care. This must include principles and knowledge relating to immunology, nutrition, physiology, etc."*

Further in Health promotion and illness prevention GMC mentions:

> *"Newly qualified doctors must be able to apply the principles, methods and knowledge of population health and the improvement of health and sustainable healthcare to medical practice.*
>
> *They must be able to:*
> *Discuss the role and impact of nutrition to the health of individual patients and societies".*

Breast feeding is the start of nutrition, the best nutrition, & the start should be on best & sound scientific footing. Focused specific approach is desirable. "Currently there is no published data on the inclusion of breastfeeding education within the UK medical school curriculum" [47]. *Biggs et al* (2020) cross-sectional study in UK has suggested that UK medical schools are not adequately preparing students to support breastfeeding patients. Further studies should explore the competency of doctors to meet the needs of lactating women, and design optimal training for UK medical students. In this study, overall, 93% (381/411) students requested further breastfeeding education [47].

Taylor & Bell (2017) have commented that high quality training in breastfeeding during medical education is historically varied. The process of becoming a board-certified physician entails more than 20 years of education. Medical school and residency training timelines and courses are relatively standardized across the United States and even internationally, but breastfeeding education varies greatly across schools and programs [48]. In view of all this and given all the evidence of benefits of breast feeding, it should be a consistent essential component in all future training, as:

"Learned practices & policies for correct start of life with

Medical education rationalization,

Benefits immediate, short term, & long-term scientific basis foundation,

Basic & advanced competencies worldwide acceleration,

For holistic health & wonderful wellbeing facilitation"

7. Conclusion

Advancing on universal health coverage vision is required. For this, it is important that right things are taught to all mothers for feeding their babies, encouraging and enabling all, for the best start of life. For breastfeeding leaving out a single or even a few mothers are undesirable and the results of this can be unpardonable. Universal health coverage is not a one-time effort, and if we are not able to implement a scientifically proven natural intervention, breastfeeding, for its full period, then it is also not universal health coverage. Our efforts should be for Universal health coverage with the new meaning – "Cover all and cover completely", a much refined and more rigorous approach [49].

"Be early to start, Be exclusive for first half of first year,

Be comprehensive with complementary feeding while also carrying on breastfeeding"

This is for all, for full recommended duration, for child's full development, and

Leading to fulfillment of development goals"

Specific initiatives are definitely needed for the health of children so that they achieve their full growth potential [50]. We need to build health systems that can monitor the continued implementation of our scientific recommendations. This calls for continued efforts by all healthcare workers, unremitting and unrelenting. We should partner all in eliminating gross health inequalities and enhancing human welfare. Scientific evidence regarding the feeding of these most vulnerable age groups has revealed clear-cut policies for implementation, which should be done with precision and perfection.

We look forward to continued cooperation with renewed vigor and vitality from all the Paediatricians and health care providers for Able, Bold, & Confident mothers, & attaining the Sustainable Development Goals, for which optimum breast and complementary feeding practices are the most important and imperative. Methodical medical education will ensure all this.

"Breastfeeding is the firm foundation & is for favorable future, hence

Comprehensive policies & complete practice,

Wonderfully with,

Medical education for supportive, sophisticated & skilled doctors"

Acknowledgements

Thankful to the formulators of all regulatory policies and guidelines and to the authors of the references quoted.

Funding

Nil.

Conflict of interest

"The authors declare no conflict of interest."

Author details

Sunil Jain[1*], Arvind Singh Kushwaha[2] and Vishal Marwaha[3]

1 Department of Paediatrics, Military Hospital Secunderabad, Telangana State, India

2 All India Institute of Medical Sciences, Nagpur, India

3 School of Medicine, Amrita Institute of Medical Sciences and Research Centre, Amrita Vishwa Vidyapeetham, India

*Address all correspondence to: sunil_jain700@rediff.com

References

[1] Victora CG, Bahl R, Barros AJD, Franca GVA, Horton S, Krasevac J, et al. Breastfeeding in the 21st century: Epidemiology, mechanisms, and lifelong effect. The Lancet. 2016;**387**(10017):475-490

[2] Victora CG, Horta BL, Loret de Mola C, Quevedo L, Pinheiro RT, Gigante DP, et al. Association between breastfeeding and intelligence, educational attainment, and income at 30 years of age: A prospective birth cohort study from Brazil. The Lancet Global Health. 2015;**3**(4):e199-e205

[3] UNICEF. 'The State of the World's Children 2016: A Fair Chance for Every Child'. Available from: www.unicef.org [Accessed: 2022-01-02]

[4] Blyth R, Creedy DK, Dennis CL, Moyle W, Pratt J, De Vries SM. Effect of maternal confidence on breastfeeding duration: An application of breastfeeding self-efficacy theory. Birth. 2002;**29**(4):278-284. DOI: 10.1046/j.1523-536x.2002.00202.x

[5] WHO. Continuing support for infant and young child feeding. In: WHO, editor. Infant and Young Child Feeding: Model Chapter for Textbooks for Medical Students and Allied Health Professionals. Switzerland: WHO Press; 2009. pp. 37-50

[6] Mother's Health. Infant and Young Child Feeding: Model Chapter for Textbooks for Medical Students and Allied Health Professionals. Switzerland: WHO Press; 2009. pp. 77-80

[7] WHO. Management and support of infant feeding in maternity facilities. In: WHO, editor. Infant and Young Child Feeding: Model Chapter for Textbooks for Medical Students and Allied Health Professionals. Switzerland: WHO Press; 2009. pp. 29-35

[8] WHO. Evidence for the Ten Steps to Successful Breastfeeding. Geneva: World Health Organization; 1998

[9] Kramer MS, Chalmers B, Hodnett ED, et al. Promotion of Breastfeeding Intervention Trial (PROBIT): A randomized trial in the Republic of Belarus. Journal of the American Medical Association. 2001;**285**(4):413-420

[10] World Health Organization. Ten Steps to Successful Breastfeeding (revised 2018). Available from: https://apps.who.int/nutrition/bfhi/ten-steps/en/index.html [Accessed: 2022-01-02]

[11] Milinco M, Cattaneo A, Macaluso A, et al. Prevalence of breastfeeding in a baby-friendly pediatric practice in Trieste, Italy: Follow up to 36 months of age. International Breastfeeding Journal. 2021;**16**:93

[12] Milinco M, Travan L, Cattaneo A, et al. Effectiveness of biological nurturing on early breastfeeding problems: A randomized controlled trial. International Breastfeeding Journal. 2020;**15**:21

[13] Raj VK, Plichta SB. The role of social support in breastfeeding promotion: A literature review. Journal of Human Lactation. 1998;**14**(1):41-45. DOI: 10.1177/089033449801400114

[14] Kearney MH. Identifying psychosocial obstacles to breastfeeding success. Journal of Obstetric, Gynecologic & Neonatal Nursing. 1988;**17**(2):98-105. DOI: 10.1111/j.1552-6909.1988.tb00519.x

[15] WHO. Report of the WHO Consultation on Birth Spacing: 13-15

June 2005. Geneva: World Health Organization; 2006

[16] Lawrence RA, Lawrence RM. Reproductive function during lactation. In: Breastfeeding: A Guide for the Medical Profession. 7th ed. Maryland Heights, Missouri: Elsevier Mosby; 2011. pp. 664-688

[17] Breastfeeding Challenges: ACOG Committee Opinion, Number 820. Obstetrics and Gynecology. 2021;**137**(2):e42-e53. DOI: 10.1097/AOG.0000000000004253

[18] Haroon S, Das JK, Salam RA, et al. Breastfeeding promotion interventions and breastfeeding practices: A systematic review. BMC Public Health. 2013;**13**:S20

[19] Aneja S. Integrated Management of Newborn and Childhood Illness (IMNCI) Strategy and its Implementation in Real Life Situation. Indian Journal of Pediatrics. 2019;**86**(7):622-627. DOI: 10.1007/s12098-019-02870-2

[20] Goldberg NM, Adams E. Supplementary water for breast-fed babies in a hot and dry climate—not really a necessity. Archives of Disease in Childhood. 1983;**58**:73-74

[21] Maternity Benefits Act 1961. Available from: http://www.ilo.org/dyn/travail/docs/678/Maternity%20Benefits%20Act%201961.pdf [Accessed 2022-01-03]

[22] Bold & Breastfeeding. The Times of India. 22 Nov 2021. Available at: https://timesofindia.indiatimes.com/india/bold-and-breastfeeding/articleshow/87830909.cms. [Accessed 2022-01-21]

[23] Horta BL, Bahl R, Martines JC, Victora CG, & WHO. Evidence on the long-term effects of breastfeeding: Systematic review and meta-analyses. World Health Organization. 2013. Available from: https://apps.who.int/iris/handle/10665/43623 [Accessed: 2022-01-26]

[24] Babakazo P, Donnen P, Akilimali P, Ali NM, Okitolonda E. Predictors of discontinuing exclusive breastfeeding before six months among mothers in Kinshasa: A prospective study. International Breastfeeding Journal. 2015;**10**:19

[25] WHO. Protecting, Promoting and Supporting Breastfeeding in Facilities Providing Maternity and Newborn Services. Geneva: World Health Organization; 2017

[26] Rollins N, Doherty T. Improving breastfeeding practices at scale. The Lancet Global Health. 2019;**7**(3):e292-e293. DOI: 10.1016/S2214-109X(18)30557-6

[27] Cresswell JA, Ganaba R, Sarrassat S, et al. The effect of the Alive & Thrive initiative on exclusive breastfeeding in rural Burkina Faso: A repeated cross-sectional cluster randomised controlled trial. The Lancet Global Health. 2019;**7**:e357-e365

[28] Wilson JC. Using Social Media for Breastfeeding Support. Nursing for Women's Health. 2020;**24**(5):332-343. DOI: 10.1016/j.nwh.2020.07.003

[29] Hurst N. Puopolo KM. Breastfeeding and maternal medications. In: Eichenwald EC, Hansen AR, Martin CR, Stark AR, editors. Cloherty & Stark's Manual of Neonatal Care. 8th edition. Philadelphia: Lippincott Williams & Wilkins: 2016.p 286-296. https://lww.com/Cloherty-and-Stark-s-Manual-of-Neonatal-Care/p/9781496343611 [Accessed 2022-01-22]

[30] Henderson G, Anthony MY, McGuire W. Formula milk versus

maternal breast milk for feeding preterm or low birth weight infants. Cochrane Database of Systematic Reviews. 2007;**4**:CD002972

[31] Polberger SKT, Raiha NCR. Individualized fortification of human milk for very low birth weight infants: Milk protein and energy analyses for improved nutritional management. Pediatric Research. 1995;**37**:316A

[32] Gribble KD. Mental health, attachment and breastfeeding: Implications for adopted children and their mothers. International Breastfeeding Journal. 2006;**1**:5

[33] Biervliet FP, Maguiness SD, Hay DM, Killick SR, Atkin SL. Induction of lactation in the intended mother of a surrogate pregnancy: Case report. Human Reproduction. 2001;**16**(3):581-583

[34] Farhadi R, Philip RK. Induction of lactation in the biological mother after gestational surrogacy of twins: A novel approach and review of literature. Breastfeeding Medicine. 2017;**12**(6):373-376. DOI: 10.1089/bfm.2016.0112

[35] Zingler E, Amato AA, Zanatta A, Vogt MFB, Wanderley MS, Neto CM, et al. Lactation induction in a commissioned mother by surrogacy: Effects on prolactin levels, milk secretion and mother satisfaction. Revista Brasileira de Ginecologia e Obstetrícia. 2017;**39**(02):86-89

[36] Bryant CA. Nursing the adopted infant. Journal of American Board of Family Medicine. 2006;**19**(4):374-379. DOI: 10.3122/jabfm.19.4.374

[37] Kushwaha AS. Newborn care in India: A crying need of the hour. Medical Journal of Armed Forces India. 2011;**67**(2):104-105

[38] United Nations. Work of the Statistical Commission pertaining to the 2030 Agenda for Sustainable Development, Resolution adopted by the General Assembly on 6 July 2017. 71/313: Available from: https://ggim.un.org/documents/a_res_71_313.pdf [Accessed: 2022-01-26]

[39] Breastfeeding: Achieving the new normal. Lancet. 2016;**387**(10017):404. DOI: 10.1016/S0140-6736(16)00210-5

[40] Rollins NC, Bhandari N, Hajeebhoy N, Horton S, Lutter CK, Martines JC, et al. Why invest, and what it will take to improve breastfeeding practices? The Lancet. 2016;**387**(10017):491-504

[41] Fewtrell MS. The long-term benefits of having been breastfed. Paediatrics and Child Health. 2004;**14**(2):97-103

[42] Sinha B, Chowdhury R, Sankar MJ, Martines J, Taneja S, Mazumder S, et al. Interventions to improve breastfeeding outcomes: A systematic review and meta-analysis. Acta Paediatrica. 2015;**104**(467):114-134. DOI: 10.1111/apa.13127

[43] Jain S, Dewey RS. The role of "Special Clinics" in imparting clinical skills: Medical education for competence and sophistication. Advances in Medical Education and Practice. 2021;**12**:513-518. DOI: 10.2147/AMEP.S306214

[44] Office of the Surgeon General (US); Centers for Disease Control and Prevention (US); Office on Women's Health (US). The Surgeon General's Call to Action to Support Breastfeeding. Rockville (MD): Office of the Surgeon General (US); 2011. Available from: http://www.surgeongeneral.gov [Accessed 2022-01-23]

[45] Medical Council of India. Competency based undergraduate

curriculum for the Indian Medical Graduate. 2018;**2**:154-155

[46] General Medical Council. Outcomes for graduates 2018. Available from: https://www.gmc-uk.org/education/standards-guidance-and-curricula/standards -and-outcomes/outcomes-for-graduates/outcomes-for-graduates# [Accessed 2022-01-23]

[47] Biggs KV, Fidler KJ, Shenker NS, et al. Are the doctors of the future ready to support breastfeeding? A cross-sectional study in the UK. International Breastfeeding Journal. 2020;**15**(1):46

[48] Taylor JS, Bell E. Medical education and leadership in breastfeeding medicine. Breastfeeding Medicine. 2017;**12**(8):476-478

[49] Jain S, Thapar RK, Gupta RK. Complete coverage and covering completely: Breast feeding & complementary feeding: Knowledge, attitude, & practices of mothers. Medical Journal of Armed Forces India. 2018;**74**(1):28-32

[50] Jain S, Thapar RK, Mallick A, Tiwari S, Yokesh D, Abhijit YV. Evidence based focused approach for fulfillment of aims: Experiences of an asthma clinic. Indian Journal of Child Health. 2017;**4**(2):170-175

Section 2

Infant Feeding in Developing Countries

Chapter 2

Infant and Young Child Feeding in the Developed and Developing Countries

Enos Mirembe Masereka, Clement Munguiko, Alex Tumusiime and Linda Grace Alanyo

Abstract

Infant feeding challenges continue to manifest in developed and developing countries. Worldwide, more than 80% of babies are breastfed in the first few weeks of birth. However, about 37%, 25%, and less than 1% are exclusively breastfed at 6 months of age in Africa, the United States of America, and the United Kingdom, respectively. These statistics are far below the World Health Organization targets of 50% and 70% by 2025 and 2030, respectively. Complementary feeding practices are varied as well due to nonadherence to Infant and Young Child Feeding (IYCF) guidelines among parents. This accounts for the current trends in malnutrition in children under–5 years of age, adolescents, and the youth, and leads to intergeneration malnutrition. In this chapter we have included sections on appropriate infant feeding; including how to initiate breastfeeding in the first hour of birth, how to exclusively breastfeed infants until 6 months of age, how to complement breastfeeding after 6 months of infant's age as well as continuing to breastfeed until 24 months of age and even beyond. Furthermore, we have included a description of how mothers who are unable to breastfeed can feed their infants on expressed breastmilk or replace breastmilk with appropriate homemade or commercial formula. This chapter as well covers infant feeding in prematurity.

Keywords: breastfeeding, diet, feeding, infant, nutrition, young child

1. Introduction

Infant feeding challenges continue to manifest in both developed and developing countries across the world. For instance, in the United States, of the 84.1% who started breastfeeding in 2017, only 25% were exclusively breastfed at 6 months of age [1]. In the UK, the percentage is even less than 1% for infants exclusively breastfed at 6 months [2]. In Sub-Saharan Africa, only 37% of infants aged less than 6 months are exclusively breastfed [3]. This is even less in South Africa and Uganda with 32% and 36%, respectively [4, 5]. Most countries are still far away from the World Health Organization (WHO) set targets of ensuring that at least 50% and 70% of infants are exclusively breastfed by 2025 and 2030, respectively [6–8]. Complementary feeding practices after 6 months of age have continued to vary due to nonadherence to Infant and Young Child Feeding (IYCF) guidelines. Only 40.1% and 32% of mothers are adherent to complementary feeding guidelines in Uganda and South Africa, respectively [4, 9]. This contributes to inappropriate infant feeding and high levels of malnutrition. For instance, the rates of stunting in South Africa and Uganda are 27% and 44.9%, respectively, for children below 5 years of age [4, 10, 11]. Infant feeding practices determine the nutrition, health, survival, growth, and development of children. It also determines the intellectual ability, quality of future citizens, social-economic transformation, and development of a country. Optimal infant feeding is recommended to achieve a healthy and economically able future generation. Optimal infant feeding includes initiation of breastfeeding within 1 h of birth, usually referred to as the golden hour, followed by active exclusive breastfeeding up to 6 months of age, unless advised otherwise by a qualified health worker. This is followed by another important age from 6 to 24 months and beyond in which breastfeeding is complemented with other foods. However, due to the risk of transmitting HIV to the infant through breastfeeding, HIV-positive mothers who have adhered to their Antiretroviral drugs (ARVs) are encouraged to breastfeed for 1 year [12]; this includes exclusive breastfeeding for the first 6 months, followed by complementary feeding up to 1 year of age. This is thought to reduce the risk of severe malnutrition among infants as well as minimize the risk of Mother to Child Transmission (MTCT). Mothers who do not wish to breastfeed can replace breastfeeding with an Affordable, Feasible, Accessible, Sustainable, and Safe (AFASS) breastfeeding substitute. Mixed feeding has been associated with a high risk for malnutrition and MTCT of HIV among HIV-exposed infants. In a study, Ogbo found that, despite this guide, infant feeding practices are varied across countries resulting in childhood illnesses, such as diarrhea [13]. This has led to poor nutritional outcomes, morbidity, and mortality among children under 5 years of age, as well as contributing to intergenerational malnutrition. Consequently, infant, childhood, and adolescent growth has been tremendously affected. The situation is more critical when it comes to the girl child; malnutrition in the girl child adversely affects the development of reproductive organs, thus increasing the risk of these young girls getting obstetric complications during labor and delivery at a later age. Poor nutritional status during early adolescent development has been cited as one of the indirect contributing factors to high maternal morbidity and mortality in developing countries. Additionally, poor nutrition contributes to poor intellectual ability. This has implications on the ability to perform in school and consequently impacts negatively on women's education and socioeconomic empowerment.

2. Initiation of breastfeeding after birth

Breast milk is the most nutritious food for a newborn and infants below 6 months of age. Initiation of breastfeeding within the first hour of birth ensures that the newborn receives colostrum or the first milk that is rich in nutrients and immunological factors [14]. Colostrum is richer in bioactive components with immune-enhancing properties. These include immunoglobulins, lactoferrin, leukocytes, lysozymes, alfa-lactalbumin, and beta-lactoglobulin compared to mature milk. Immunoglobulin A (IgA) is the most abundant and IgM and IgG antibodies are in lower concentrations in breast milk. These confer protection against infection before the infant's natural immune system is built. IgA coats and seals a baby's respiratory and intestinal tract to prevent germs, such as bacteria, viruses, fungi, and parasites from entering the body and bloodstream. IgG is involved in the prevention of autoimmune and allergic diseases during childhood [15]. Despite the benefits of early initiation of breastfeeding, only 58.3% of mothers initiate breastfeeding within 1 h of birth in Sub-Saharan Africa with a huge variation between countries, ranging from 24 to 86% [16]. Immediately after the baby is born, the midwife places the baby on the mother's abdomen. The baby is dried, stimulated to breathe, and then is placed onto the mother's chest with the baby's mouth closer to the mother's breasts. Normally the baby shows signs that he or she wants to breastfeed called breastfeeding readiness cues, as they are commonly referred to, are then recognized by the mother or caregiver. These may include mouthing—frequently opening the mouth and leaking the lips, rooting—moving the mouth toward whatever touches the baby's cheeks, sucking—attempts to suckle whenever the baby's mouth or lips touches anything, and hand to mouth or hand to hand movements. If the baby's mouth is not wide open, the mother or other caretaker should bring the nipple to touch the baby's cheeks, the baby then moves the mouth toward the nipple and opens the mouth. The mother should then support the breast and put the nipple and areolar into the wide open mouth of the baby. The baby will then spontaneously start to suckle. Mothers with big breasts will need to support the breast for the baby, those with small breasts may only be required to position the baby in close proximity to the breast during the time when the mother is still lying on her back and the baby is lying skin to skin during the third stage of labor. When the baby becomes hungry and is not given the breast, she or he shows the breastfeeding readiness cues, and when giving the breast is further delayed, it will make the baby vigorously cry and will be irritable. All mothers should be supported to initiate and establish breastfeeding as soon as possible after birth and preferably within the first hour after childbirth. Breastfeeding within the first hour after birth has very profound benefits. It will result in an early and sustained breastmilk production by the mother as well as help in shortening the third stage of labor. After birth, the reduction in progesterone and estrogen following the expulsion of the placenta triggers the prolactin reflex and its increased production from the anterior pituitary gland. Further production of prolactin is stimulated when the baby continues to suckle the breast [17] (**Figure 1**). This ensures that the breast is full of breast milk and adequate for the infant.

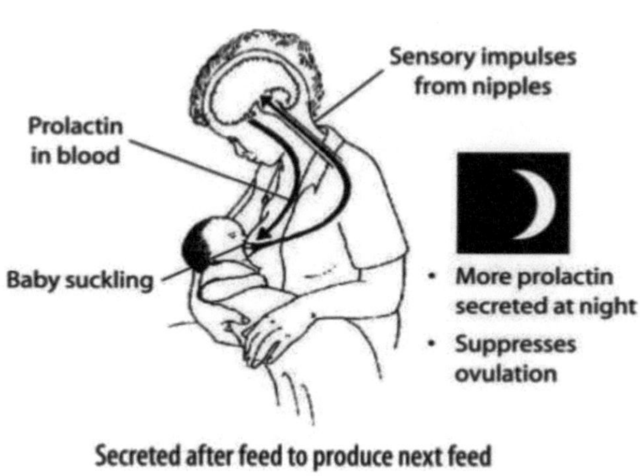

Figure 1.
Prolactin reflex.

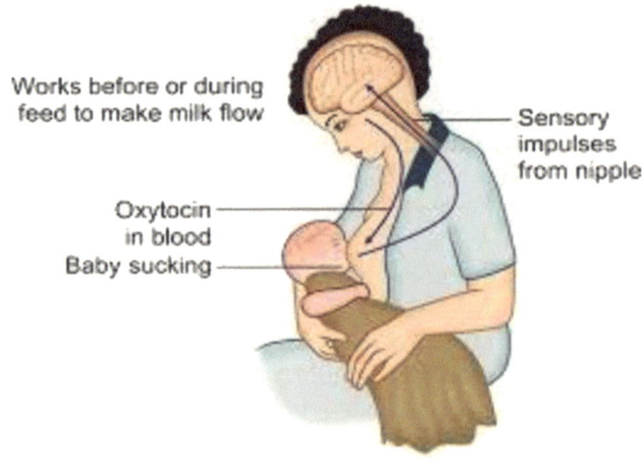

Figure 2.
Oxytocin reflex.

Suckling the breast stimulates oxytocin from the posterior pituitary [17]. Oxytocin is responsible for milk ejection or let-down reflex (**Figure 2**). Oxytocin causes the myoepithelium of the breast to contract, this causes the temporarily stored breastmilk to be released from the lactiferous ducts and ampulla, out through the pores of the nipple, and into the baby's mouth.

Milk ejection or let-down reflex can be triggered by suckling, thoughts, sights, sounds, or odors that a mother associates with her baby (**Figure 3**). In each of these cases, neurohumoral reflex leads to a burst of prolactin secretion as well as stimulation of the oxytocin reflex. Breastfeeding mothers should ensure that the breast is emptied on each breastfeeding occasion and should breastfeed at least every 2–3 h. The more frequently and thoroughly the breasts are emptied, the faster they will refill with breastmilk.

Immediately after childbirth, breast milk may not be present except for a small amount of colostrum, this may be troublesome for mothers with babies demanding to breastfeed and may lead to the introduction of pre-lacteal feeds, a practice that reduces

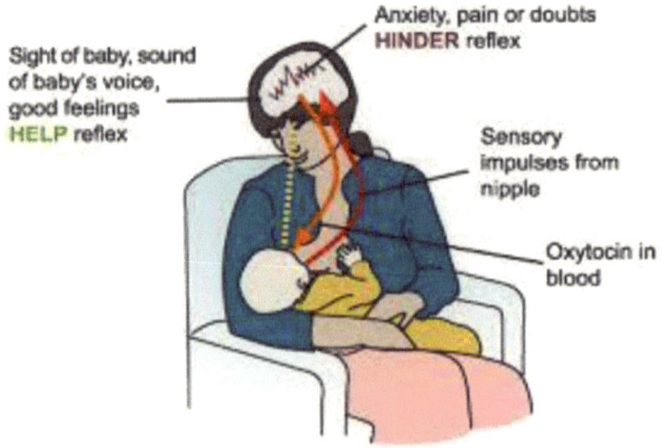

Figure 3.
Helping and hindering factors for the oxytocin reflex.

suckling frequency and reduces the amount of breastmilk. Mothers should be made aware that breast milk may fully appear in 1–7 days and average on the third day for most mothers depending on the frequency of breastfeeding, nutrition status, psychological status, especially anxiety and physical health of the mother. Mothers who deliver by caesarian section are less likely compared to their counterparts who deliver vaginally to initiate breastfeeding in the first 1 h of delivery [18]. This is due to the fact that mothers delivering by cesarean section will spend extra time (30 min to 1 h or more) in the theater as the operation is being concluded and during this time, the mother may not be in contact with the baby. In addition, mothers who are delivered by caesarian section usually have high anxiety levels and pain that hinder oxytocin reflex (**Figure 3**). Such mothers need extra support to ensure the early initiation of breastfeeding. Obstetric and medical complications associated with pregnancy, labor, and delivery that may delay breastfeeding should be anticipated, prevented, or managed early to reduce on the delay of breastfeeding [19, 20]. Mothers should be encouraged to breastfeed as early as when able for adequate breastmilk production. Each mother should receive instruction, assistance, and support in positioning and ensuring proper attachment on the breast until she is able to do so independently. Recommended techniques used to attach babies to breasts are discussed in this chapter later.

3. Exclusive breastfeeding

Exclusive breastfeeding is defined as giving only breast milk to the infant, without mixing it with water, other liquids, herbal preparations, or food in the first 6 months of life with the exception of vitamins, mineral supplements, or medicines. Exclusive breastfeeding during the first 6 months provides all the required nutrients to the baby. Offers protection against childhood illnesses, such as diarrhea and pneumonia. It leads to better physical growth, neuro-development, and increases intelligence [21]. In HIV-exposed infants, exclusive breastfeeding, in addition, offers protection against severe acute malnutrition, diarrhea, and even death [22]. Under normal circumstances, an infant should be exclusively breastfed for the first 6 months of life. Although this is associated with great benefits, the practice is still poor and in sub-Saharan Africa, only 36% of mothers exclusively breastfeed [23]. The mother should breastfeed every 2 h for a total of 8–12 times or more during day and night. However, mothers should learn to breastfeed every time the baby demands and may stimulate the baby to breastfeed if the baby does not demand the breast beyond 2 h. For successful exclusive breastfeeding, mothers should learn to position the baby and ensure appropriate attachment of the baby to the breast. Good baby positioning and attachment facilitate adequate breastfeeding. It ensures that both baby and mother are comfortable, the baby suckles optimally until the breast is emptied and he or she gets satisfied. There are some exceptional situations where the length of breastfeeding may be shortened. For instance, there are times when some babies at the age of 4 or 5 months may not be satisfied by breast milk alone. This may be due to unmodifiable factors, such as inadequate breastmilk production from the mother. A baby with a high body weight may also not be satisfied by breast milk alone at this age bracket despite all attempts to improve the quantity produced by the mother. In these special circumstances, other feeds may be introduced in the fourth or fifth months. Also, if the mother or baby has other illnesses other than HIV that makes the baby unable to exclusive breastfeeding for 6 months, other feeds may be introduced earlier. In such special circumstances, mothers are strongly advised to consult a qualified professional health worker for advice before such other feeds are introduced. It is, therefore, imperative to also know how other feeds should be introduced to the baby's feeding practices. This topic is also elaborately discussed in this chapter later.

4. Attachment to the breast and baby positioning

Another important aspect of active and effective breastfeeding practice is how to attach and position the baby onto the breast. Good attachment to the breast is

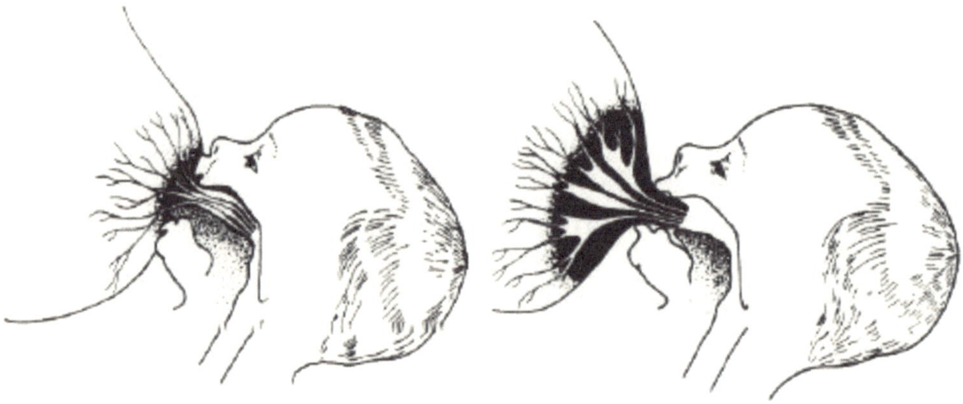

Figure 4.
Good and poor attachment to the breast.

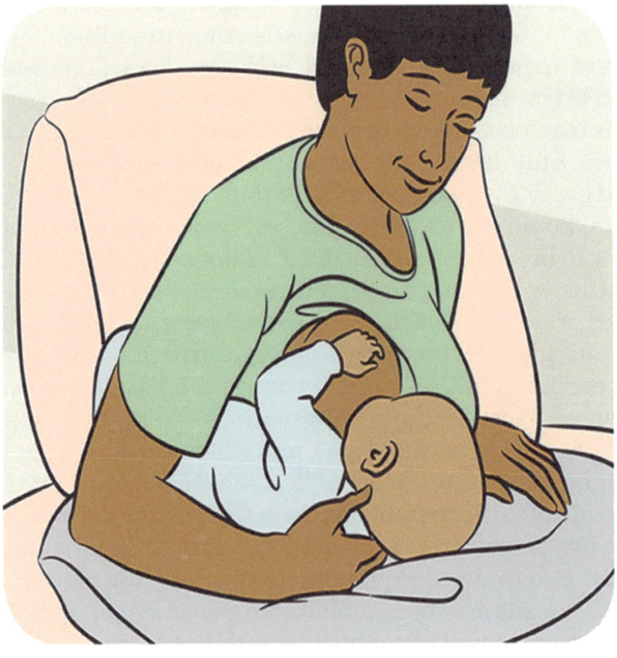

Figure 5.
Underarm position.

DOI: http://dx.doi.org/10.5772/intechopen.103012

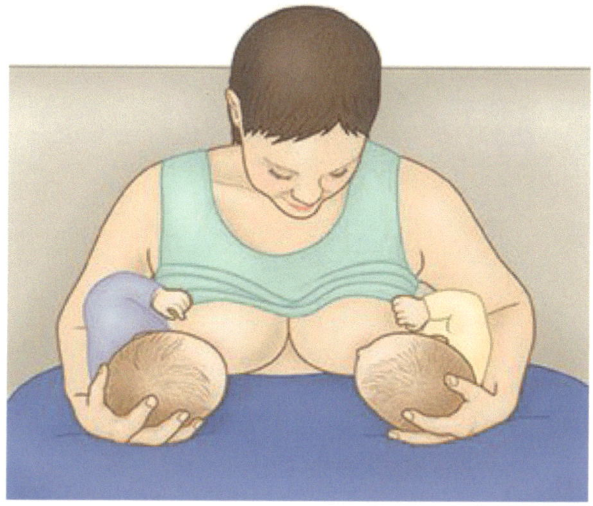

Figure 6.
Underarm position for twins.

necessary for effective suckling. The baby is well attached when he or she has taken much of the areola and the underlying tissues into his or her mouth, and the lower lip is turned outward (**Figure 4**). This attachment enables the baby to suckle adequately, fill the cheeks with breastmilk, and consequently swallow the milk well. Poor attachment may result in painful nipples, breast engorgement, less breastmilk production, unsatisfied baby, frustrated baby, and failure to thrive or gain weight.

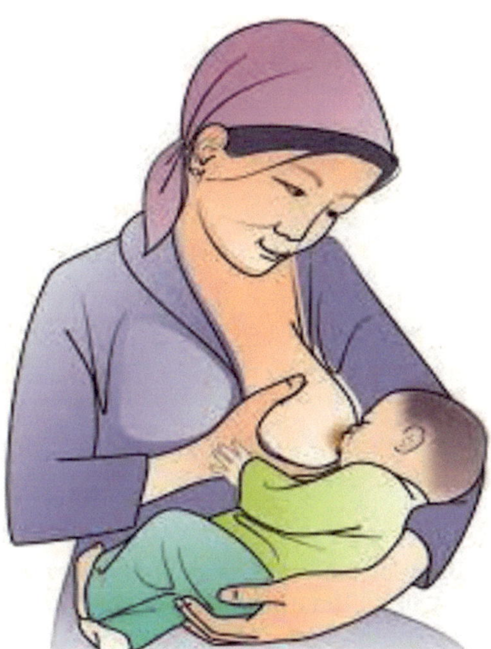

Figure 7.
Cradle position.

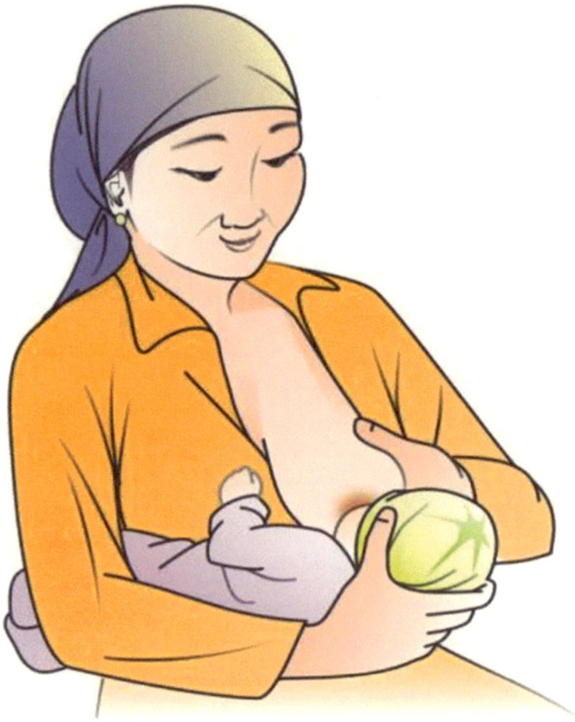

Figure 8.
Cross cradle position.

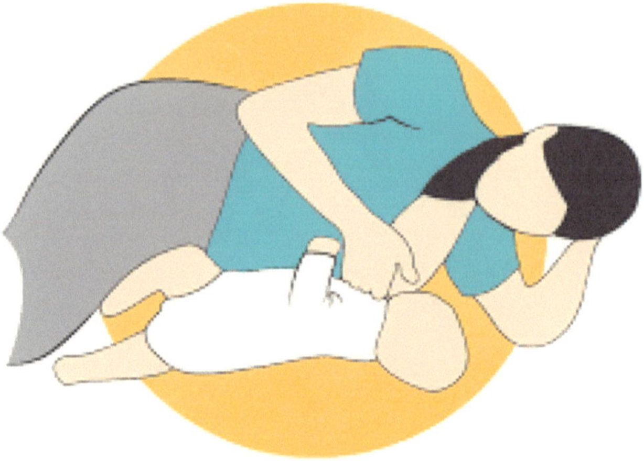

Figure 9.
Side lying position.

Baby positioning entails steps the mother should follow to hold the baby and ensure that the baby reaches the breast without strain and the mother breastfeeds comfortably while relaxed. The baby position adopted by the mother may vary depending on whether the mother is seated, lying, has a small versus big baby, or is nursing twins. The different positions include; cradle baby position or hold, underarm position,

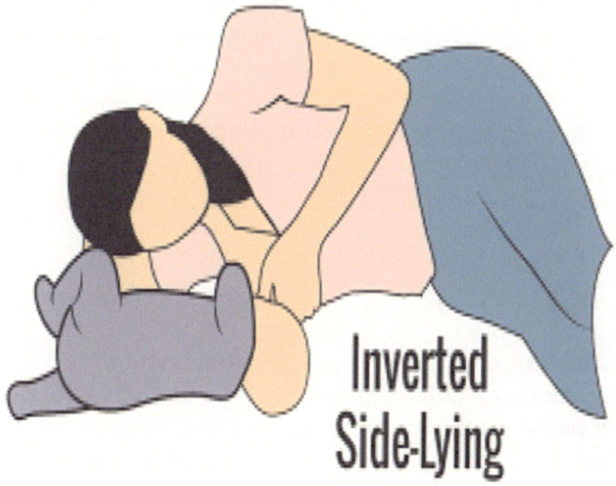

Figure 10.
Inverted side lying position.

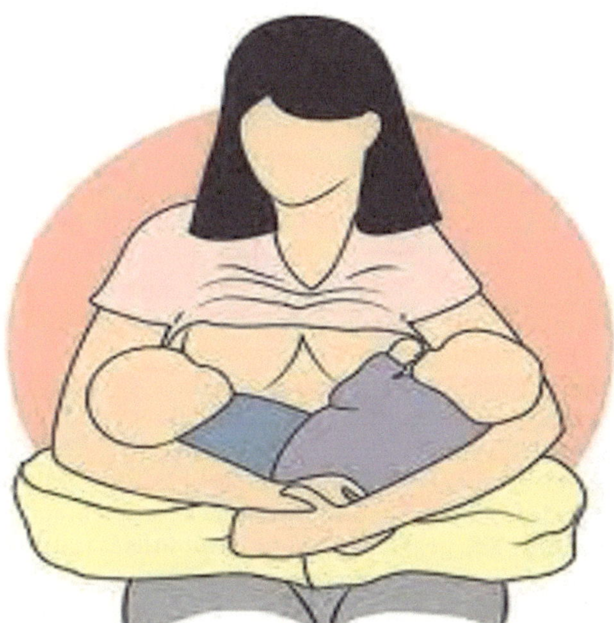

Figure 11.
Cross position for twins.

cross-cradle, lying down, underarm position for twins, and cross position for twins (**Figures 5–11**). In each of these, mothers should note the four key points, which are as follows:

a. The baby's body should be inline: A baby cannot suckle or swallow easily if his head is twisted or bent.

b. The baby is held close to the mother's body: A baby cannot attach well to the breast if he or she is far away from it. The baby's whole body should almost face his or her mother's body.

c. The baby is well supported: The baby's whole body is supported with the mother's arm along the baby's back. This is particularly important for newborns and young babies. For older babies, support from the upper part of the body is usually enough.

d. Placing the *baby on the breast* with the *nose* at the level of *nipple* will encourage him or her to open the mouth wide and attach to the *breast* well.

Many mothers in developing countries know and commonly use cradle and side-lying breastfeeding positions. This leaves some mothers with no other options yet there are other positions that can be used for the comfort of the mother and the satisfaction of the baby. It is advisable to use various breastfeeding positions depending on the mother's comfort.

5. Complementary feeding and weaning practices

Complementary feeding is the feeding of the baby with other foods in addition to breastfeeding at 6 months of age when breastmilk alone is no longer adequate to meet the nutritional needs of the infant. In Sub-Saharan Africa, infant feeding is characterized by either early or late introduction of complementary feeds. In a study, 59% of mothers introduced other feeds early and 30.7% did not receive other foods between 6 and 8 months of infant's age [24]. Additional foods should be introduced into the infant's diet at 6 months of age and continued until breastfeeding is entirely stopped at 24 months of age or beyond if the mother so wishes to extend breastfeeding. Weaning is the process of stopping the infant from breastfeeding. Weaning should be done gradually; however, it may be done abruptly in HIV-positive mothers at 1 year of infant's age to reduce the risk of transmitting HIV to the infant. HIV-positive mothers who are well retained in HIV care and are adhering well to Highly Active Antiretroviral Therapy (HAART) are encouraged to breastfeed at least for the first 1 year of age [25, 26]. In 1 year, the mother exclusively breastfeeds for 6 months and introduces complementary feeds after 6 months of infant's age. The period from 6 to 24 months is critical and includes rapid growth and development. Due to this, the energy requirement doubles and other nutrient deficiencies are common if complementary feeds are not appropriately introduced as recommended (**Figures 12–15**).

Infants require adequate caloric intake to provide energy for growth and physical activity. The energy requirement increases with age. For example, at age < 3 months (3.5–5 kg), the energy requirement is 110 Kcal/kg/day (450–550 kcal); at age 3–5 months (5.5–7 kg), the energy requirement is 100 Kcal/kg/day (550–700 kcal); at age 6–8 months (8–9 kg), the energy requirement is 95 Kcal/kg/day (700–800 kcal) and age 9 months–1 year (9–10 kg), the energy requirement is 100 Kcal/kg/day (900–1000 kcal) (**Figure 12**). To fill the gap, the infant should be fed on energy rich and thick foods, such as porridge, banana (matooke), cassava, and Irish potato, from 6 to 24 months of age. This may be supplemented with cooking oil, ghee, and other sources of energy.

DOI: http://dx.doi.org/10.5772/intechopen.103012

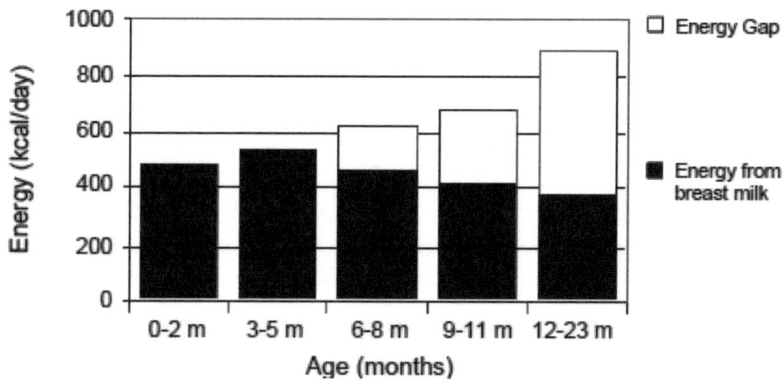

Figure 12.
Energy requirement by age and amount supplied by breastmilk.

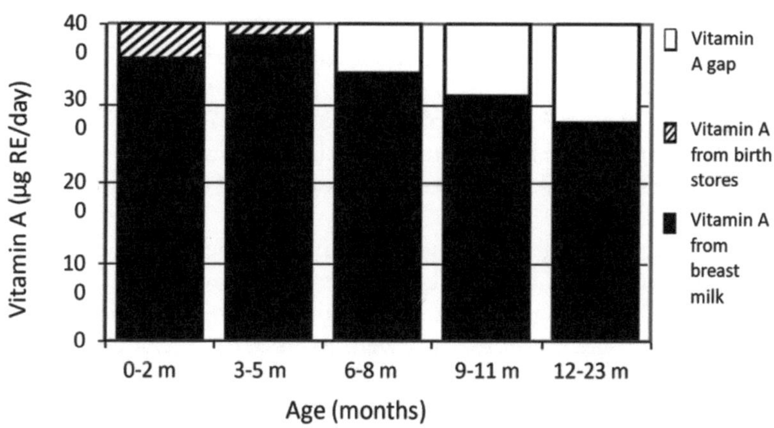

Figure 13.
Vitamin a requirement by age and amount supplied by breastmilk.

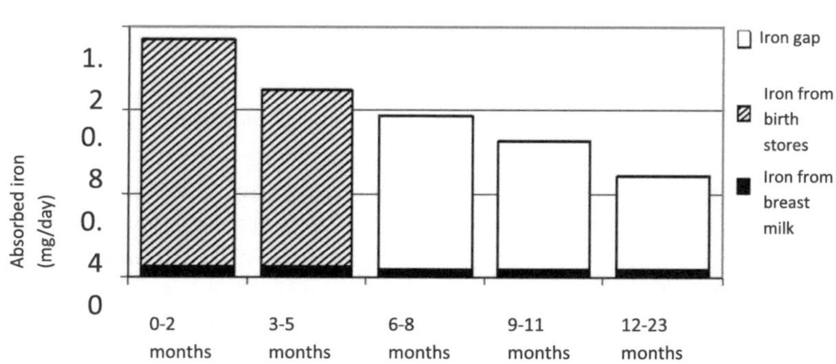

Figure 14.
Iron requirement by age and amount supplied by breastmilk.

To fill the vitamin-A gap at 6 months of age, as shown in **Figure 13**, the infant's diet should be supplemented with dark-green leaves and yellow-colored fruits and vegetables, such as dodo, pumpkin, carrot, papaya, spinach, and mangoes.

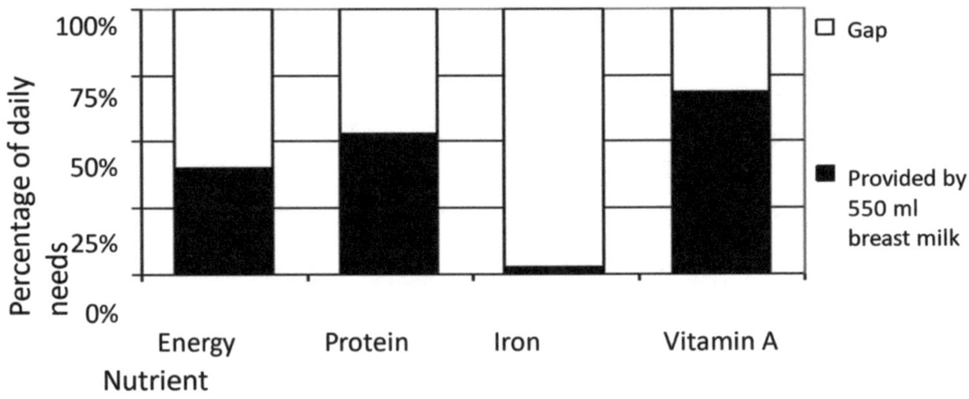

Figure 15.
Summary of gaps to be filled by complementary foods for a 12–23-month-old child.

To fill the iron gap at 6 months of age, as shown in **Figure 14**, the infant's diet should be supplemented with millet, dark leafy green vegetables, liver, poultry, and eggs.

To fill the protein gap, at 6 months of age, as shown in **Figure 15**, the infant's diet should be supplemented with both animal and plant sources of proteins. Animal sources include; chicken, eggs, fish, meet, and milk. Plant sources include; beans, groundnuts, and peas.

To meet all the nutritional requirements, infants should receive nutritionally adequate and safe complementary foods while continuing to breastfeed for up to 24 months or beyond. Starting other foods in addition to breastmilk at 6 completed months of age can help the infant to grow well. After 6 months of age, infants should be fed on thick porridge and mashed foods. Mashed foods should include major nutrient ingredients, such as carbohydrates, proteins, fats, and vitamins in rightful proportions. Mineral requirements are met by giving water and micronutrient supplements to the infant during feeding. It is important for parents to understand that complementary feeds should be timely, meaning that they should be introduced at appropriate infant age; they should be adequate both in nutrient variability and quantity; they should be safe. Foods should be well prepared, hygienic, well stored, and fed using clean hands and utensils. Additionally, parents should desist from using bottles and teats to feed their infants and instead use a cup and a spoon. This is because bottles and teats are difficult to clean and keep hygienic by many parents. Parents should feed infants in consistence with a child's signals of appetite and satiety and the meal frequency and feeding should be suitable for age. Parents should take care in the feeding of infants by being responsive to the infant's clues for hunger and also encourage the infant to eat, especially those that have reached the age for feeding themselves. There is variability in the zeal or enthusiasm to feed self across infants; those that are poor at feeding themselves will need additional support and encouragement from parents or caregiver. Feeding the child should take an active form. Children should be actively supported during feeding. They should be actively fed by adults and not by their fellow young ones. Each child should have his or her food on a separate serving plate. Parents or caregivers should not feed many children of varying age groups on the same plate. Feeding many children on the same plate, some children will be out-competed and will not be satisfied. In addition, in case the food served on the plate is eaten to completion, more food should be added and the child encouraged to continue feeding until the child is satisfied and some food is left on the serving plate. World Health Organization (WHO) and the Ministry of Health (MoH) recommend that infants should initially receive complementary foods 2–3 times a day between 6 and 8 months, increase to 3–4 times daily between 9 and 11 months, and 12–24 months of age [27]. Additional nutritious snacks should also be offered 1–2 times per day for ages 12–24 months of age. Parents should gradually increase food thickness and variety as the infant gets older, adapting to the infant's requirements and abilities. Infants can eat soft mashed and semi-solid foods beginning at 6 months, by 8 months most infants can eat more solid foods. By 12 months, most infants can eat the same types of foods as consumed by the rest of the family while keeping in mind the need for nutrient-dense foods including animal-sourced foods like meat, poultry, fish, eggs, and dairy products. Parents should avoid foods in a form that may cause chokings, such as whole grapes, or raw carrots. Avoid giving drinks with low nutrient value, such as tea, coffee, and sugary soft drinks. Parents should limit the amount of juice offered to avoid displacing more nutrient-rich foods.

6. Replacement feeding practice

This refers to feeding an infant who is not breastfeeding with a diet that provides all the nutrients that the infant needs. This may be applicable in mothers who may not wish to breastfeed as in HIV-positive mothers or if a mother dies immediately after childbirth and the baby survives. Other circumstances in which breastfeeding may be contraindicated, the mother may not express breastmilk and should replace breastfeeding include; metabolic disease, such as galactosemia of the infant, the mother is taking chemotherapeutic agents, the mother is infected with human T-cell lymphotropic virus type I or type II, the mother is using an illicit street drug, such as cocaine, the mother has suspected or confirmed Ebola virus disease. Conditions in which the mother may temporarily replace breastfeeding and may not express breastmilk include; the mother is infected with untreated brucellosis, the mother is taking certain medications, vaccinations, drugs, tobacco, and alcohol, the mother is undergoing diagnostic imaging, the mother has an active herpes simplex virus (HSV) infection with lesions present on the breast and other bilateral breast diseases. Conditions in which the mother should temporarily not breastfeed, but can express breastmilk include; the mother has untreated active tuberculosis (the mother may resume breastfeeding once she has been treated appropriately for 2 weeks and is documented to be no longer contagious), the mother has active varicella (chickenpox) infection that developed within the 5 days prior to delivery to the 2 days following delivery [28–30]. The breastmilk substitute should be a suitable substitute for breastmilk, such as a commercial or homemade formula. However, parents should be aware that available substitutes may not wholly replace the benefits of breastfeeding and breastfeeding remains the most appropriate mode of feeding infants 0–6 months of age. Selected replacement feeds should meet the AFASS criteria; that is to say, they should be Acceptable—the mother perceives no significant cultural or social barriers to replacement feeding. Feasible—the mother has adequate knowledge, skills, resources, and support to correctly mix, formula or milk, and feed the infant up to 12 times in 24 h. Affordable—the mother and family can pay the costs of, replacement feeding associated with fuel, clean water, and all ingredients without compromising the health and nutrition, of the family. Sustainable—the mother has access to a continuous and uninterrupted supply of all ingredients needed for safe replacement feeding as long as the infant needs it. Safe—replacement feeds are correctly and hygienically stored, prepared, and fed in nutritionally adequate amounts. The infant is fed with clean hands and preferably by the cup.

6.1 Homemade formula

Homemade formulas are made from local foods available at home. While preparing a local formula, mothers should include at least one type of food from each of the following classes. (a) Sources of proteins, such as beans, peas, groundnuts, milk, meat, chicken, fish, and eggs; (b) sources of carbohydrates, such as millet flour, sorghum flour, maize flour, potatoes, and matooke or banana; (c) sources of vitamins, such as dodo, nakatti, buga, tomato, eggplant and carrot, and sources of fats, such as ghee, shea butter, margarine, and palm oil in their rightful proportions.

6.1.1 Home-modified formula for infants 0–6 months of age

Infants who are not breastfed from birth can be given a homemade milk-based formula prepared from cow's, goat's, camel's, sheep's, or buffalo's milk. Such formula can be prepared as follows;

1. Fresh cow's, goat's, or camel milk

   a. 40 ml milk +20 ml water +4 g sugar = 60 ml

   b. 60 ml milk +30 ml water +6 g sugar = 90 ml

   c. 80 ml milk +40 ml water +8 g sugar = 120 ml

   d. 100 ml milk +50 ml water +10 g sugar = 150 ml

2. Sheep and Buffalo milk

   a. 30 ml milk +30 ml water +3 g sugar = 60 ml

   b. 45 ml milk +45 ml water +5 g sugar = 90 ml

   c. 60 ml milk +60 ml water +6 g sugar = 120 ml

   d. 75 ml milk +75 ml water +8 g sugar = 150 ml

Micronutrient supplements should be given with all the above home-prepared infant formulas; this includes minerals, such as manganese—7.5 μg, Iron—1.5 mg, copper—100 μg, zinc—205 μg and iodine, and vitamins, such as vitamin A—300 IU, vitamin D—50 IU, vitamin E—1 IU, vitamin C—10 mg, vitamin B1—50 μg, vitamin B2—80 μg, Niacin—300 μg, vitamin B6—40 μg, folic acid—5 μg, Pantothenic acid—400 μg, vitamin B12—0.2 μg, vitamin K—5 μg, and biotin—2 μg.

6.1.2 Home-modified complementary formula for infants 6 months of age and above

Home-modified complementary formula can be made of porridge as a major source of energy, mixed with pounded roasted groundnuts or ground nuts paste as a major source of protein, mixed with pounded dodo as a major source of vitamin, mixed with margarine as a supplementary source of energy. The thickness of the preparation should be regulated based on the age of the infant and the ability of the infant to eat. Other sources of energy, proteins, vitamins, and fats can as well be used depending on availability.

6.2 Commercial formulas

Commercial infant formulas are designed to resemble human milk as closely as possible, although none has ever duplicated it. The exact composition of infant formula varies with the manufacturer but all must meet specific standards. Four main categories of commercially prepared formulas; cow's milk-based formula such as NAN (milk-based with iron), soy-based formulas—commonly used for children who are lactose or cow's milk intolerant, such as Soy Isomil infant formula and Enfamil ProSobee *Infant Formula*, casein or whey-hydrolysate formulas—used primarily for children who cannot tolerate the other two formulas, and amino acid formulas—used for infants with multiple food protein intolerances.

It is important for parents to note that commercially available infant feeding formulas occur in two categories. That is to say; those prepared for infants 0–6 months of age, for example, NAN for 0–6 months infants and those prepared for infants 6–12 months of age for example NAN for infants 6–12 months of age. This is because nutrient requirements vary at different ages of infants.

Commercial formulas are available in three forms: 1. Ready-to-feed formula- is the most expensive but easiest to use. 2. Concentrated formula- is less expensive than ready to feed, it is diluted with equal parts of water and can be stored in the refrigerator for 48 h after opening. 3. Powdered formula—is the least expensive, it is easily mixed by using one scoop of 60 ml for every 60 ml of water or one scoop of 30 ml for every 30mls of water. It is important to bear in mind the quantity of feed required depending on the infant's age.

6.3 Feeding the child using formula feeds

The first feeding of the formula is ideally given after the neonate's initial transition to extrauterine life. At birth, the baby's stomach is very small with a cherry-like size and volume capacity of about 20mls. In the first 24 to 48 h of life, a newborn will typically consume 15–30 ml of formula at each feeding. Intake gradually increases during the first week of life, most newborns are taking 90–150 ml at each feeding by the end of the second week or sooner. The newborn infant should be fed at least every 3–4 h, even if waking the newborn is required for the feeding. However, usually rigid feeding schedules are not recommended. Most newborns need six to eight feedings in 24 h and the number of feedings decreases as the infant matures and consumes more at each feeding. During feeding, parents are encouraged to sit comfortably, holding the infant closely in a semi-upright position with good head support. Feeding provides an opportunity to bond with the baby through touching, talking, and singing to the infant.

6.4 Preparation of powdered infant formula

According to the World Health Organization, parents using formula feeds should follow the following steps to prepare and feed their infants [31];

a. Wash your hands with soap and water and dry using a clean cloth.

b. Wash all feeding and preparation equipment thoroughly in hot soapy water. Use a clean bottle and teat brush to scrub the inside and outside of bottles and teats to make sure that all remaining feed is removed from the hard-to-reach places.

c. Rinse thoroughly in safe water.

d. Fill a large pan with water.

e. Place the cleaned feeding and preparation equipment into the water. Make sure that the equipment is completely covered with water and no air bubbles are trapped.

f. Cover the pan with a lid and bring to a rolling boil, making sure the pan does not boil dry.

g. Keep the pan covered until the feeding equipment is needed.

h. Clean and disinfect a surface on which to prepare the feed.

i. Wash your hands with soap and water, and dry with a clean or disposable cloth.

j. Boil some safe water. If using an automatic kettle, wait until the kettle switches off. If using a pan to boil water, make sure the water comes to a rolling boil.

k. Read the instructions on the formula's packaging to find out how much water and how much powder you need. Adding more or less formula than instructed could make infants ill.

l. Taking care to avoid scalds, pour the correct amount of boiled water (which has been allowed to cool to no less than 70°C) into a cleaned and sterilized feeding cup. Use a clean, sterile thermometer to check the temperature.

m. Add the exact amount of formula to the water in the feeding cup.

n. Mix thoroughly by stirring with a cleaned and sterilized spoon.

o. Immediately cool to feeding temperature by holding the feeding cup under cold running tap water, or by placing it in a container of cold or iced water. So that you do not contaminate the feed, make sure that the level of the cooling water is below the top of the cup.

p. Dry the outside of the cup with a clean or disposable cloth.

q. Label the cup with information, such as formula type, infant's name or ID, date and time made, and preparer's name.

r. Check the temperature of the feed by dripping a little onto the inside of your wrist. It should feel lukewarm, not hot. If it still feels hot, cool some more before feeding.

s. Feed infant.

t. Throw away any feed that has not been consumed within two hours.

For parents using the bottle for feeding their infants, the bottle should be held so that fluid fills the nipple and none of the air in the bottle is allowed to enter the nipple. The bottles, nipples, rings, and caps should be washed in warm soapy water, using a bottle and nipple brush to facilitate thorough cleaning. They should be placed in boiling water for 5 min and allowed to air dry, this should be done at least prior to the first use and thereafter unless they are cleaned in the dishwasher. However, due to difficulties associated with maintaining the hygiene of bottles, nipples, rings, and caps, parents are strongly advised to feed their infants using a cup and a spoon as described later in this chapter.

7. Infant and young child feeding in the context of HIV/AIDS

It is estimated that 20% of all Mother-To-Child-Transmission (MTCT) cases occur through infants acquiring HIV from their HIV-positive mothers after birth through breastfeeding [32]. However, with option-B plus, this risk is eliminated. According to the consolidated guidelines for prevention and treatment of HIV in Uganda, all HIV exposed infants should be exclusively breastfed for the first 6 months of age irrespective of HIV status [33]. Meanwhile, the infant's first Polymerase Chain Reaction (PCR) test should be taken at 6 weeks of age. The mother continues to be on HAART and exclusive breastfeeding. Complementary foods should be introduced at 6 months of age. The second PCR should be done at 9 months of age, 3 months following the introduction of complementary foods. If the infant remains HIV negative, the mother continues to breastfeed until the infant is 1 year of age after which the infant should entirely feed on family foods as discussed later in this chapter. The third PCR test should be done at 6 weeks after caseation of breastfeeding. For infants found to be HIV infected, the infant should be breastfed as per the general population until the infant is 24 months old and beyond. On the other hand, if the mother does not wish to breastfeed and Infant is HIV negative, the mother can consider discontinuing breastfeeding as early as possible and use replacement feeding if Affordable, Feasible, Acceptable, Sustainable, and Safe (AFASS).

7.1 Feeding HIV-negative infants (12: 24 months) of HIV-positive mothers

Mothers who are HIV positive and have babies with a negative second PCR at 9 months, will cease breastfeeding at 12 months of infant's age [33]. The mother will adopt alternative infant feeding options as described earlier under formula feeding. The third PCR will be taken at 6 weeks after cessation of breastfeeding and an HIV antibody test at 18 months of age. The Alternative forms of infant feeding will include other forms of milk such as cow's or goat's milk; of at least 500 ml (one cup) a day. In addition, the mother will continue to feed the infant 5 times a day, which includes three main meals of nutritious foods from locally available foods and two extra snacks.

8. Feeding a child (2: 6 years)

It is important to encourage mothers to give a variety of foods prepared from the family meal (each meal should consist of carbohydrate, protein, vegetables) at least 3 main meals a day. Encourage caregivers to give nutritious snacks between meals, such as fruit (banana, pawpaw, orange, and mangoes), an egg, bread, enriched thick porridge, or a glass of milk. Sick and improving infants and children should be fed on small, frequent meals that include porridge enriched with milk or groundnut paste, margarine, honey, oil, cooked skinned mashed beans, thickened soups, and many more others to aid quick recovery.

9. Common problems of breastfeeding

Breastfeeding problems cause difficulty in breastfeeding. May also cause insufficient breastmilk production, failure of the mother to give the breast to the infant, frustration of the infant, discontinuation of breastfeeding, and failure to thrive. These include breast engorgement, sore nipples, plugged or clogged milk ducts, mastitis, and insufficient or decreased milk production.

9.1 Breast engorgement

Breast engorgement is caused by overfilling of the breast due to infrequent or ineffective emptying of the breast [34]. It occurs around the 3rd–5th day postpartum. This condition is characterized by vascular congestion, increased vascularity, accumulation of milk in the breast tissue, and edema related to swelling and obstruction of lymphatic drainage. The breast is usually painful and tender on palpation, firm, and hot. The breast may appear shiny and the nipples may flatten. Management requires breastfeeding more frequently (every 2 h), massaging the breast as the baby breastfeeds, breastfeeding on one breast until it softens before changing to another one, cold compress may relieve swelling, expressing breastmilk may be done if the baby does not empty the breast completely, Non-Steroidal Anti-Inflammatory Drugs (NSAIDS) may be prescribed to relieve pain, a warm water birth before breastfeeding and use of cabbage leaves (put in a fridge and applied) may be helpful.

9.2 Sore nipple

Nipples may be tender, cracked, or bleeding due to poor attachment or poor latch-on, sucking, and monilial infection. Sore nipple causes pain during breastfeeding and thus disrupts infant feeding. The prevention and management involve correct positioning and attachment to the breast. To make the nipple less painful, the mother should first express some milk to moisten the nipple. If pain continues, the mother should check for proper breast–baby attachment. If pain continues, the mother should stop breastfeeding for a few minutes and start again, and should ensure that the baby's mouth is widely open for both the nipple and areola to enter. If pain continues, the mother should check for the presence of a short frenulum. If present, it should surgically be released. If both nipples have sores, the mother may breastfeed on the breast with a less sore nipple first followed by the more painful one. It is most important to clean the nipple with water after breastfeeding and also to express some milk and spread it around the nipple to air dry. The mother should be advised to expose the nipple to the air as much as possible. She may apply purified lanolin cream to prevent further abrasion after breastfeeding. Antibiotics creams may be applied if nipples are extensively cracked. Other un-approved creams are not recommended.

9.3 Plugged or clogged milk ducts

Plugging of milk ducts is due to poor feeding, delayed or missed feeding. It is important to apply a warm compress to the affected area, this may promote the emptying and release of the plug. Breastfeeding more frequently is preferred and while breastfeeding, the baby should begin with the affected breast to ensure emptying.

9.4 Mastitis

Mastitis is the inflammation of the breast [35, 36]. It is usually caused by staphylococcus, streptococcus, and Escherichia coli (E-coli). The condition presents with fever, chills, body aches, and headache initially. On examination, the breast is tender, warm and reddened. It is caused by poor breast hygiene, inadequate emptying of the breast during breastfeeding, plugged ducts, sudden decrease in number of feedings, abrupt weaning, and cracked nipples. Management includes administration of antibiotics (penicillins or cephalosporins plus metronidazole) for 10–14 days, NSAIDS for the pain and inflammation can be prescribed, warm compress to relieve pain, and emptying of the breast while breastfeeding. If the breast cannot be emptied by breastfeeding, the mother is encouraged to express the remaining breastmilk. The mother should have enough rest, take plenty of oral fluids, and a balanced diet. In case of a breast abscess, surgical intervention is required.

9.5 Insufficient or decreased milk production

Insufficient milk production is one of the biggest challenges faced by mothers currently [37]. It can result from any of the following causes; insufficient glandular tissue-some women may not have enough milk-making ducts to meet the baby's needs, endocrine problems, such as hypo or hyperthyroidism, hormonal contraceptive methods, previous breast surgery—for either cosmetic or medical reasons reduces breast ducts and create scarring within the breast, taking medications or herbs containing anti prolactin agents, such as bromocriptine, pseudoephedrine, and methergine, sucking difficulties-due to poor attachment, not feeding at night—women who do not breastfeed at night may produce less breastmilk because prolactin hormone is higher at night, scheduling feedings—infrequent breastfeeding such as in working women may make the breast to be full for a long time and this leads to a reduction in milk secretion, birth jaundice or birth medications—medications for epidural anesthesia may affect baby's breastfeeding for close to a month. Jaundice may make the infant sleepier and not able to breastfeed, supplementation—when breastfeeding is supplemented, the baby becomes satisfied soon and may not breastfeed to empty the breast. When less breastmilk is removed through breastfeeding, less is produced by the breast leading to low breastmilk production. Lastly, the nutritional status, psychological and physical health of a mother plays a significant role in breastmilk production. Mothers who are breastfeeding should eat a well-balanced diet, take plenty of fluid, be psychosocially supported and be free from illness for adequate breastmilk to be produced.

9.6 Measures to correct insufficient breastmilk

Every breastfeeding woman's wish is to produce adequate breastmilk for the baby. This can be achieved through ensuring good maternal nutrition, good maternal psychological and physical health, breastfeeding at least 2-hourly and on both breasts for 12–20 min or until breasts are empty, good breast attachment, avoiding medications that interfere with lactation, treating endocrine disorders that may interfere with breastmilk production, always breastfeeding at night, stopping hormonal birth control offenders, managing jaundice if any and stopping or avoiding unjustified infant feeding supplementation.

10. Breastfeeding and working

Working women usually face difficulties breastfeeding their infants, especially after their maternity leave. Maternity leave is short (3 months), especially in Uganda. At 3 months of age, the mother is still required to exclusively breastfeed and the infant does not feed on any other feeds except breastfeeding. Some working conditions may not favor some mothers to fulfill this obligation. If such mothers are not supported, they are left with no choice other than to opt for mixed feeding, breastfeeding supplementation, or for replacement feeding. Breastmilk produced becomes less and does not meet the baby's nutritional requirements resulting in malnutrition. Mothers who fall in such category may be advised on appropriate replacement feeding if they are able to fulfill the AFASS criteria or else express breastmilk and employ someone else to feed the baby using a cup.

10.1 Expressing breastmilk

Expressing breastmilk may be necessary especially when a mother goes to work and leaves the baby at home. It may also be necessary to feed a baby who is too weak and cannot breastfeed such as those who are ill and those with low birth weight. Other situations include a baby who cannot latch on due to an inverted nipple, breast engorgement. All mothers should learn how to express their milk so that they know what to do if the need arises. Breast milk can be stored for about 8 h at room temperature or up to 24 h in a refrigerator.

10.2 How to express breastmilk by hand

The woman should sit comfortably and upright. She should prepare a clean dry container for Expressed Breastmilk (EBM); she can use a cup, glass, jug, or jar with a wide mouth. She should hold the container near her breast. Put her thumb on her breast above the nipple and areola, and her first finger on. The breast below the nipple and areola, opposite the thumb. She supports the breast with her other fingers. Press her thumb and first finger slightly inwards toward the chest wall. She should avoid pressing too far or she may block the milk ducts. The mother should press her breast behind the nipple and areola between her finger and thumb. She should press on the larger ducts beneath the areola. Press and release, press and release.

At first, no milk may come, but after pressing it a few times, milk starts to drip out. It may flow in streams if the oxytocin reflex is active. The mother should press the areola in the same way from the sides to make sure that milk is expressed from all segments of the breast. Avoid rubbing or sliding her fingers along the skin. The movement of the fingers should be more like rolling. Avoid squeezing the nipple itself. Pressing or pulling the nipple cannot express the milk. It is the same as the baby sucking only the nipple.

The mother should express one breast for at least 3–5 min until the flow slows; then express the other side; and then repeat both sides. She can use either hand for either breast and change when they tire. The mother should express the breast milk adequately over 20–30 min, especially in the first few days when only a little milk may be produced. Express as often as the baby would breastfeed. This should be at least every 3 h, including during the night. If she expresses only a few times, or if there are long intervals between expressions, she may not be able to produce enough milk.

10.3 How to stimulate oxytocin reflex

Help the mother psychologically by reducing any sources of pain or anxiety, sitting quietly and privately or with a supportive friend, and holding her baby with skin-to-skin contact if possible. The mother can be assisted to hold her baby on her lap while she expresses herself, warm her breasts by applying a warm compress, or warm water, or have a warm shower. She can also be told to stimulate her nipples, and massage or stroke her breasts lightly. The helper can rub her back.

10.4 How to store expressed breastmilk

Choose a suitable container made of glass or plastic that can be kept covered. Clean it by washing in hot soapy water, and rinsing in hot clear water. If the mother is hand expressing, she can express directly into the container. If storing several containers, each container should be labeled with the date. The mother should use the oldest milk first. The baby should consume expressed milk as soon as possible after expression. Feeding of fresh milk (rather than frozen) is encouraged. Frozen breastmilk may be thawed (unfrozen) slowly in a refrigerator and used within 24 h. It can be defrosted by standing in a jug of warm water and used within one hour, as it is warm. The mother should not boil milk or heat it in a microwave as this destroys some of its properties and can burn the baby's mouth.

Fresh breast milk should be stored at 25–37°C for 4 h, at 15–25°C for 8 h, and below 15°C for 24 h. Milk should not be stored above 37°C. Refrigerated (2–4°C) milk can be stored for up to 8 days. Frozen Breast Milk can be kept in a freezer compartment inside the refrigerator for 2 weeks. If milk is put in a freezer part of a refrigerator (freezer), it can be kept for a period of 3 months, and if in a separate deep freeze, it can stay for a period of 6 months. To de-freeze or warm breast milk, do not freeze for 24 h or place the container in warm water to thaw quickly.

10.5 Feeding EBM to a baby using a cup

Wash your hands. Put breastmilk into a small cup, approximately 60 mls. Hold the baby on your lap in a sitting upright or semi-upright position, the baby should not lie down too much. Hold the small cup or glass to the baby's lips. Tip it so that the water just reaches the lips, the edges of the cup touch the outer part of the baby's upper lip, and the cup rests lightly on his lower lip. This is normal when a person drinks. At this point, a real baby becomes quite alert and opens his mouth and eyes. He makes movements with his mouth and face, and he starts to take the milk into his mouth with his tongue. Babies older than about 36 weeks gestation try to suck. Some milk may spill from the baby's mouth. You may want to put a cloth on the baby's front to protect his clothes. Spilling is commoner with babies of more than about 36 weeks gestation, and less common with smaller babies. Do not pour the milk into a baby's mouth; just hold the cup to his lips. When a baby has had enough, he closes his mouth and will not take any more of this feed. If he has not taken the calculated amount, he may take more next time, or he may need feeds more often. Measure his intake over 24 h, not just at each feed.

10.6 How much should a baby take in 24 hours?

Babies who weigh 2.5 kg or more can take 150 ml milk per kg body weight per day. Divide the total into eight feeds, and give 3-hourly. Babies who weigh less than 2.5 kg (Low-birth-weight); start with 60 ml/kg body weight. Increase the total volume by 20 ml per kg per day, until the baby is taking a total of 200 ml per kg per day. Divide the total into 8–12 feeds, to feed every 2–3 h. Continue until the baby weighs 1800 g or more, and is fully breastfeeding. Check the baby's 24-hour intake. The size of individual feeds may vary. If the baby was previously receiving other milk, reduce the amounts of other milk gradually as the breast milk production goes up. It is normal for the amount of milk that a baby takes at each feed to vary, whatever the method of feeding, including breastfeeding. Babies feeding by cup may take more or less than the calculated amount. If possible, offer a little extra, but let the baby decide when to stop. If a baby takes a very small feed, offer extra at the next feed, or give the next feed early, especially if the baby shows signs of hunger. Low-birth-weight (LBW) babies need only very small volumes during the early days. If the mother can express even a small amount of colostrum, it is often all that her baby needs.

11. Feeding the premature babies

A premature baby is one who is born alive before 37 weeks of pregnancy are completed. In other terms, this baby is usually referred to as one born too soon. Factors that are associated with preterm labor that later result in preterm baby include infections, multiple pregnancies, maternal diseases, and conditions such as diabetes, hypertension, or incompetent cervix. Other factors may be maternal abdominal trauma and at times, pregnancies are terminated prematurely on medical grounds to save the life of the mother. However, in some cases, the cause of preterm birth is not known. Preterm babies are usually classified as extreme preterm, very preterm, and moderate preterm. Extreme preterm babies are those who are born before 28 weeks of pregnancy, very preterm ones are those born between 28 and 32 weeks and moderate ones are those delivered between 32 and 37 weeks. About 15 million preterm babies are born annually worldwide, representing a global preterm birth rate of about 11% [38]. Of these, over 60% of preterm births occur in Africa and South Asia [38]. According to the WHO report, 12% of babies are born too soon compared with 9% in higher-income countries [38].

About one million preterm babies die due to preterm birth before age of 5 years, and this accounts for about 18% of all deaths among children under 5 years. Preterm deaths are highest in low- and middle-income countries especially those that are in South East Asia and Sub-Saharan Africa [38]. The challenge of preterm birth and death is worth to be squarely addressed if countries are to achieve Sustainable Development Goal 3 number 3.2 that aims at ending all the preventable deaths of newborn babies and children aged under 5 years by 2030. The common causes of preterm death are complications usually associated with feeding, breathing, body temperature, and infections. Preterm babies usually have feeding problems because their gastrointestinal system and accessory muscles are not yet well developed. They may not be able to coordinate sucking, swallowing, and breathing. They may not be able to take enough volume of milk from the breast before tiring due to weak muscle tone. Premature babies have a long neck that provides little support for the jaw, weak sensation around the mouth, slow and incomplete root, and gag reflexes. They have incompetence of the lower esophageal sphincter, have delayed gastric emptying, and decreased intestinal motility that may affect feeding tolerance. Preterm babies are also more likely to have feeding challenges because of impaired rectal sphincter reflex which can cause a delay in evacuating stool. There are other important considerations that may cause nutritional deficiencies. Preterm babies usually have a high growth rate and metabolic needs that require additional nutritional requirements. Premature babies also have inadequate nutritional stores and poorly developed physiological systems. Many times, preterm babies also suffer from various illnesses such as infections which as well increase nutritional demands [39].

Survival rates of preterm infants can greatly improve if the emphasis is put on optimizing nutritional demands. The goals of feeding in preterm babies are three-fold—(i) to meet the nutritional requirements of the baby, (ii) to prevent feeding-related complications, especially Necrotizing Enterocolitis (NEC), and (iii) to optimize short- and long-term growth outcomes. In view of all above, it is usually advisable that the feeding abilities of all premature babies based on many factors, such as age, weight, and clinical status be assessed shortly after birth by a qualified health worker. The health worker will provide nutritional support to the mother or caretaker depending on the findings and the diagnosis.

American Academy of Pediatrics recommends the use of human milk for premature babies as the enteral feeding choice. In addition to nutritional values, human breast milk provides premature babies with immunological defense, hormones, and enzymes that are essential to growth and development. The smaller the preterm baby, the higher the nutritional demand, and the longer fortification of feeds will be required. It should be remembered that about 60% of total iron stores are accrued during the last trimester of pregnancy. Also, during fetal development, transfer of calcium and phosphorus from the mother to the fetus occurs in the third trimester, especially between 32 and 36 weeks of gestation. Therefore, premature babies are at higher risk of developing anemia and osteopenia. To prevent these conditions, it is recommended that their feeds are fortified with iron, calcium, and phosphorus. Usually, 2 mg per kg of iron is provided through a supplement of multivitamin for 12 months. Calcium and phosphorus supplements are also recommended as well.

If the baby has a birth weight of 1500 g or less and is stable, feeding is started with Expressed Breast Milk (EBM) of 5mls and is increased carefully by 5 mls until the baby is ready for the transition. If the baby is between 1500 g and 2000 g and is stable, then feeding can be started with 7.5 mls of EBM and is also increased according to as above. If the premature baby has a weight of more than 2000 g, 10 mls of EBM is given and is also increased steadily as explained earlier. In all cases, EBM should initially be given through a nasogastric tube because the baby may not be able to swallow effectively. However, if the baby has suckling reflexes, he/she should be progressively attached to the breast as well to stimulate sucking and swallowing. Cautious feeding then should continue as close monitoring for growth, nutritional needs, feeding, and developmental milestones.

12. Summary and conclusion

Infant feeding challenges continue to manifest in developed and developing countries. Worldwide, more than 80% of babies are breastfed in the first few weeks of birth. About 37%, 25%, and less than 1% are exclusively breastfed at 6 months of age in Africa, the United States of America, and the United Kingdom, respectively. These statistics are far below the World Health Organization targets of 50% and 70% by 2025 and 2030, respectively. Complementary feeding practices are varied as well due to nonadherence to Infant and Young Child Feeding (IYCF) guidelines among parents. This accounts for the current trends in malnutrition in children under 5 years of age, adolescents and the youth, and leads to intergeneration malnutrition. Breastfeeding is important for the proper nutrition, health, survival, growth, and development of children. This issue is more critical when it comes to the girl child. Inappropriate Infant feeding and malnutrition in the girl child adversely affect her reproductive organs, growth, and development and is one of the contributing factors to a difficult childbirth, maternal morbidity, and mortality. Malnutrition in the girl child has implications on the ability of the girl to perform in school, remain in school and consequently impacts women's education and socioeconomic empowerment. Appropriate infant feeding can be achieved if mothers can initiate breastfeeding within the first hour of birth, exclusively breastfeed their infants until 6 months of age, complement breastfeeding after 6 months with appropriate and safe complementary feeds as well as continue to breastfeed until the infant is 24 months of age and beyond. Mothers who are unable to breastfeed can feed their infants on expressed breastmilk or replace breastmilk with appropriate homemade or commercial formula as recommended. Optimal infant feeding is recommended to achieve a healthy and economically able future generation. Both global and regional innovation strategies and efforts, however, are needed to boost rates of exclusive breastfeeding as well as breastfeeding infants up to 24 months of age and even beyond.

Author details

Enos Mirembe Masereka[1*], Clement Munguiko[2], Alex Tumusiime[1] and Linda Grace Alanyo[3]

1 Department of Nursing and Midwifery, School of Medicine, Kabale University, South Western, Uganda

2 Department of Nursing, School of Health Sciences, Soroti University, Soroti, Eastern Uganda

3 Department of Nursing and Midwifery, School of Health Sciences, Mountains of the Moon University, Fort Portal, Mid-Western Uganda

*Address all correspondence to: mirembeenos@gmail.com

References

[1] Rupnicki S. Breastfeeding Report Card United States. Atlanta, Georgia, United States: CDC; 2020. Available from: https://www.cdc.gov/breastfeeding/pdf/2020-Breastfeeding-Report-Card-H.pdf?fbclid=IwAR1VWEDC9AdIcppg_DUQjSNE6yV7DWgyJB_Wo20pnADz1vAscpYPTRuUUOo

[2] McAndrew F, Thompson J, Fellows L, Large A, Speed M, Renfrew MJ. Infant feeding survey 2010. Leeds: health and social care information Centre. 2012;**2**(1):87. Available from: https://sp.ukdataservice.ac.uk/doc/7281/mrdoc/pdf/7281_ifs-uk-2010_report.pdf

[3] Victora CG, Bahl R, Barros AJ, França GV, Horton S, Krasevec J, et al. Breastfeeding in the 21st century: Epidemiology, mechanisms, and lifelong effect. The Lancet. 2016;**387**(10017):475-490. DOI: 10.1016/S0140-6736(15)01024-7

[4] Sayed N, Schönfeldt HC. A review of complementary feeding practices in South Africa. South African Journal of Clinical Nutrition. 2020;**33**(2):36-43. DOI: 10.1080/16070658.2018.1510251

[5] Nabunya P, Mubeezi R, Awor P. Prevalence of exclusive breastfeeding among mothers in the informal sector, Kampala Uganda. PLoS One. 2020;**15**(9):e0239062. DOI: 10.1371/journal.pone.0239062

[6] World Health Organization. Global Nutrition Targets 2025: Stunting Policy Brief (No. WHO/NMH/NHD/14.3). Geneva, Switzerland: World Health Organization; 2014. Available from: https://www.who.int/nutrition/publications/infantfeeding/global-bf-scorecard-2018.pdf?ua=1; https://apps.who.int/iris/bitstream/handle/10665/149022/WHO_NMH_NHD_14.7_eng.pdf; https://apps.who.int/iris/bitstream/handle/10665/149019/WHO_N?sequence=1

[7] WHO/UNICEF. The Extension of the 2025 Maternal, Infant and Young Child Nutrition Targets to 2030. New York, New York, United States. Available from: https://www.who.int/nutrition/global-target-2025/discussion-paper-extension-targets-2030.pdf: UNICEF; 2017

[8] WHO, U., & World Health Organization. The Extension of the 2025 Maternal, Infant and Young Child Nutrition Targets to 2030. Geneva: World Health Organization; 2018

[9] Aber H, Kisakye AN, Babirye JN. Adherence to complementary feeding guidelines among caregivers of children aged 6-23 months in Lamwo district, rural Uganda. Pan African Medical Journal. 2018;**31**(1):17

[10] UDHS. Uganda Demographic Health Survey. Drexel Hill, PA, United States: UDHS; 2016. p. 2016. Available from: https://dhsprogram.com/pubs/pdf/FR333/FR333.pdf

[11] Masereka EM, Kiconco A, Katsomyo E, Munguiko C. The prevalence and determinants of stunting among children 6-59 months of age in one of the sub-counties in the Rwenzori sub-region, Western Uganda. Open Journal of Nursing. 2020;**10**(03):239. DOI: 10.4236/ojn.2020.103016

[12] WHO. Updates on HIV and Infant Feeding. Geneva, Switzerland: WHO; 2016. Available from: https://apps.who.int/iris/bitstream/handle/10665/246260/9789241549707-eng.pdf;jsessionid=D5BBC4228C5509DD44BC3601B00D0180?sequence=1

[13] Ogbo FA, Agho K, Ogeleka P, Woolfenden S, Page A, Eastwood J, et al. Infant feeding practices and diarrhoea in sub-Saharan African countries with high diarrhoea mortality. PLoS One. 2017;**12**(2):e0171792. DOI: 10.1371/journal.pone.0171792

[14] Rodríguez-Camejo C, Puyol A, Fazio L, Rodríguez A, Villamil E, Andina E, et al. Antibody profile of colostrum and the effect of processing in human milk banks: Implications in immunoregulatory properties. Journal of Human Lactation. 2018;**34**(1):137-147. DOI: 10.1177/0890334417706359

[15] Palmeira P, Carneiro-Sampaio M. Immunology of breast milk. Revista da Associação Médica Brasileira. 2016;**62**(6):584-593. DOI: 10.1590/1806-9282.62.06.584

[16] Teshale AB, Tesema GA. Timely initiation of breastfeeding and associated factors among mothers having children less than two years of age in sub-Saharan Africa: A multilevel analysis using recent demographic and health surveys data. PLoS One. 2021;**16**(3):e0248976. DOI: 10.1371/journal.pone.0248976

[17] Lawrence RA. Physiology of lactation. In: Breastfeeding. Amsterdam, Netherlands: Elsevier; 2022. pp. 58-92. DOI: 10.1016/B978-0-323-68013-4.00003-1

[18] Hobbs AJ, Mannion CA, McDonald SW, Brockway M, Tough SC. The impact of caesarean section on breastfeeding initiation, duration and difficulties in the first four months postpartum. BMC Pregnancy and Childbirth. 2016;**16**(1):1-9. DOI: 10.1186/s12884-016-0876-1

[19] Taha Z, Hassan AA, Wikkeling-Scott L, Papandreou D. Factors associated with delayed initiation and cessation of breastfeeding among working mothers in Abu Dhabi, the United Arab Emirates. International Journal of Women's Health. 2021;**13**:539. DOI: 10.2147/IJWH.S303041

[20] Rukindo M, Tumwebaze M, Mijumbi EM. First hour initiation of Breast Feeding & Associated Factors, among mothers at post Natal Ward in Fort Portal referral hospital, Uganda. Open Journal of Epidemiology. 2020;**11**(01):1. DOI: 10.4236/ojepi.2021.111001

[21] Couto GR, Dias V, de Jesus Oliveira I. Benefits of exclusive breastfeeding: An integrative review. Nursing Practice Today. 2020;**7**(4):1-10. DOI: 10.18502/npt.v7i4.4034

[22] Kindra G, Coutsoudis A, Esposito F, Esterhuizen T. Breastfeeding in HIV exposed infants significantly improves child health: A prospective study. Maternal and Child Health Journal. 2012;**16**(3):632-640. DOI: 10.1007/s10995-011-0795-8

[23] Yalçin SS, Berde AS, Yalçin S. Determinants of exclusive breast feeding in sub-Saharan Africa: A multilevel approach. Paediatric and Perinatal Epidemiology. 2016;**30**(5):439-449. DOI: 10.1111/ppe.12305

[24] Gebremedhin S. Core and optional infant and young child feeding indicators in sub-Saharan Africa: A cross-sectional study. BMJ Open. 2019;**9**(2):e023238. DOI: 10.1136/bmjopen-2018-023238

[25] Thomas TK, Masaba R, Borkowf CB, Ndivo R, Zeh C, Misore A, et al. Triple-antiretroviral prophylaxis to prevent mother-to-child HIV transmission through breastfeeding—The Kisumu breastfeeding study, Kenya: A clinical trial. PLoS Medicine. 2011;**8**(3):e1001015. DOI: 10.1371/journal.pmed.1001015

[26] Samburu BM, Kimiywe J, Young SL, Wekesah FM, Wanjohi MN, Muriuki P, et al. Realities and challenges of breastfeeding policy in the context of HIV: A qualitative study on community perspectives on facilitators and barriers related to breastfeeding among HIV positive mothers in Baringo County, Kenya. International Breastfeeding Journal. 2021;**16**(1):1-13. DOI: 10.1186/s13006-021-00385-1

[27] MoH. Policy Guidelines on Infant and Young Child Feeding for Uganda 2009. Singapore: MoH; 2009. Available from: https://www.health.go.ug/docs/Policy_gl_IYCF.pdf; https://extranet.who.int/nutrition/gina/en/node/11500

[28] Davanzo R. Controversies in breastfeeding. Frontiers in Pediatrics. 2018;**6**:278. DOI: 10.3389/fped.2018.00278

[29] Mitchell KB, Johnson HM. Breast conditions in the breastfeeding mother. In: Breastfeeding. Amsterdam, Netherlands: Elsevier; 2022. pp. 572-593. DOI: 10.1016/B978-0-323-68013-4.00016-X

[30] Sattari M, Serwint JR, Levine DM. Maternal implications of breastfeeding: A review for the internist. The American Journal of Medicine. 2019;**132**(8):912-920. DOI: 10.1016/j.amjmed.2019.02.021

[31] World Health Organization. How to Prepare Powdered Infant Formula in Care Settings. Geneva, Switzerland: World Health Organization; 2007. Available from: https://www.who.int/foodsafety/publications/micro/PIF_Care_en.pdf

[32] John-Stewart G, Mbori-Ngacha D, Ekpini R, Janoff EN, Nkengasong J, Read JS, et al. Breast-feeding and transmission of HIV-1. Journal of Acquired Immune Deficiency Syndromes. 2004;**35**(2):196

[33] MoH. Consolidated guidelines for Prevention and Rreatment of HIV in Uganda (2020 Version). Singapore: MoH; 2020. Available from: http://library.health.go.ug/publications/hivaids/consolidated-guidelines-prevention-and-treatment-hiv-uganda

[34] Mangesi L, Zakarija-Grkovic I. Treatments for breast engorgement during lactation. Cochrane Database of Systematic Reviews. 2016;**6**:1-47. DOI: 10.1002/14651858.CD006946.pub3

[35] Amir LH, Trupin S, Kvist LJ. Diagnosis and treatment of mastitis in breastfeeding women. Journal of Human Lactation. 2014;**30**(1):10-13. DOI: 10.1177/0890334413516065

[36] Pevzner M, Dahan A. Mastitis while breastfeeding: Prevention, the importance of proper treatment, and potential complications. Journal of Clinical Medicine. 2020;**9**(8):2328. DOI: 10.3390/jcm9082328

[37] Kent JC, Prime DK, Garbin CP. Principles for maintaining or increasing breast milk production. Journal of Obstetric, Gynecologic & Neonatal Nursing. 2012;**41**(1):114-121. DOI: 10.1111/j.1552-6909.2011.01313.x

[38] WHO. Born too Soon: The Global Action Report on Preterm Birth. Geneva, Switzerland: WHO; 2012. Available from: https://www.who.int/pmnch/knowledge/publications/preterm_birth_report/en/index3.html

[39] Oregon Paediatric Nutrition Practice Group. Nutrition Practice Care Guidelines for Preterm infants in the Community. Seattle, WA: OPNPG; 2016. Available from: https://www.oregon.gov/oha/ph/healthypeoplefamilies/wic/documents/preterm.pdf

Chapter 3

Persistence of Chronic Childhood Undernutrition in Ecuador during a Period of Economic Growth: Exploring the Contributing Factors to This Paradox

Margarita Manosalvas

Abstract

Between 2004 and 2014 the rate of reduction of chronic childhood undernutrition (CCU) prevalence in Ecuador was about 0.2% per year, while since 1999 it was reduced to an average higher than 0.83% per year. In the same period, Ecuador experienced an economic growth of more than 4% of GDP per year on average. Commonly, child undernutrition has been assumed as the effect of a combination of a set of factors related to deprivation situations. Therefore, we are facing a paradox. The objective of this investigation is to explore this paradox. To accomplish this aim, a mixed research strategy is presented: the children's undernutrition key indicators are compared using the Surveys of Living Conditions (SLC) for the years 1999, 2006, and 2014. Changes and continuities in the relevant indicators are identified, in the next phase; the analysis of those indicators is deepened with qualitative research. Results are integrated and a plausible explanation is constructed.

Keywords: chronic childhood undernutrition, eating habits, economic growth

1. Introduction

Between 2004 and 2014, chronic childhood undernutrition (CCU) in Ecuador decreased at a rate of two-tenths per year, while since 1999 it has been reducing to an average of more than eight-tenths per year. Since 2006, not only is it evident that the reduction of the CCU slowed down but also this is a period in which the Gross Domestic Product (GDP) of the country grew to more than 4% on an annual average. It was also a period in which the National Government increased its investment in programs aimed at reducing this public health problem. If we assume that childhood undernutrition is the result of a set of physical, social, and environmental factors associated with situations of deprivation, then we are facing a paradox. The objective of this research is to identify the factors behind this paradox. Why is chronic child undernutrition reduced at a slower rate in a period of economic growth? For this, a mixed research strategy is proposed: the key indicators are compared using the Surveys of Living Conditions (SLC) for the years 1999, 2006, and 2014. Changes and continuities are identified in the relevant variables of the CCU, then, these relevant variables are explored in greater depth with qualitative research techniques. Results are integrated and a plausible explanation is constructed. The results of this research provide elements for a better understanding of the persistence of the CCU in Ecuador.

The document includes five sections: the first presents the CCU as a public problem and its indicators in the global and regional context. The second briefly presents the theoretical framework of the studies on undernutrition and the theoretical propositions on which this study is based to analyze the slowdown in the decrease of the CCU. The third part explains the mixed method followed as a research strategy for this analysis. In the fourth the results are exposed and, finally, in the fifth section, the discussion of the main findings is presented.

2. Chronic childhood undernutrition (CCU) as a public problem

According to the Global Nutrition Report, in 2015 there were 164 million stunted children in the world, this is the most commonly used indicator to determine the incidence of chronic childhood undernutrition (CCU). It is considered that 45% of all deaths of children under five are related to some type of undernutrition ([1], pp. 4).

Undernutrition in the first 1000 days from conception, entails a "waste of human potential" [2]. In these crucial days, the body is forming rapidly fundamental components for brain development and the future growth of each person. Damage caused by undernutrition in this first stage of life tends to be irreversible. Studies show that school performance of malnourished children is less than its potential under normal conditions; undernutrition leads to a lower physical and cognitive capacity in adult life. Boys and girls who suffered undernutrition in childhood are more likely to be overweight and develop chronic cardiovascular diseases, diabetes and cancer, and even mental health problems. When the girls who suffer from undernutrition are mothers probably their children will also suffer from it [2–5].

There are several types of undernutrition: underweight (low weight for age) or acute malnutrición (low weight for height), reflects changes in the short term as a result of recent disease or insufficiencies; the CCU (low height-for-age) reflects a situation of deprivation of long term that is not determined genetically but which can be transmitted intergenerationally. A longitudinal study of the Multicentre Growth Reference Study Group,[1] which included boys and girls of various ethnic groups in various countries, has shown children's same growth potential regardless of their ethnicity [7].

The way to measure the prevalence of CCU is through "anthropometry." Using protocols and surveys, the height of children under 5 years of age in a population group is measured; the value of the size is called "Z score"; through the analysis of variance, the Z scores are compared with respect to the international standard reference named "growth curves." Two standard deviations from the reference value are used as the cutoff point. The values that are below this limit indicate that the child is undernourished. The first reference curve for growth was established by the National Center for Health Statistics of the United States (NCHS) in 1978, from then countries have used this parameter to define the prevalence of chronic child undernutrition,

[1] See Ref. [6].

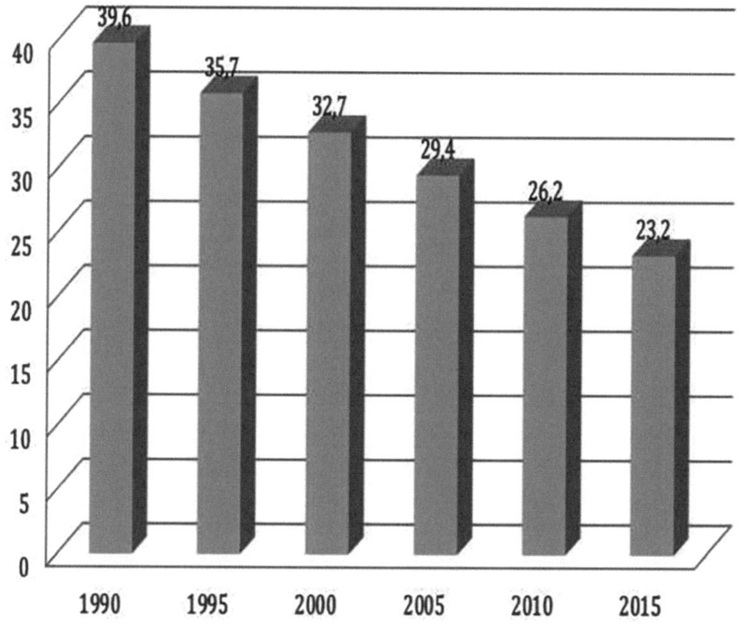

Figure 1.
Child chronic undernutrition rate worldwide. Source: with data from UNICEF [8].

understood as "low height for age." In 2006, WHO updated the referential growth curve by establishing new parameters for measurement[2] ([6], pp. 942–943). Although there are still countries using the NCHS curves of 1978. The data presented below are calculated according to the WHO standard of 2006.

According to UNICEF, the prevalence of undernutrition in the world went from close to 40% in 1990 to 23.2% in 2015, as shown in the following graph (**Figure 1**).

This represents an average annual reduction of 0.66% points. The regions that stand above the world average prevalence of chronic child undernutrition are South Asia, reaching a prevalence of 37%, and Sub-Saharan Africa with a prevalence of 35% ([2], p. 181). More than three-quarters of children with chronic child undernutrition worldwide are located in these two regions. The regions that are further away from the world average are Latin America and the Caribbean with 11%, and North America with 2% (**Figure 2**) [8].

The chronic child undernutrition rate in Latin America and the Caribbean shows a sustained reduction over time. In 1990 the prevalence was around 25% and for the

[2] In April 2006, the World Health Organization (WHO) published new standards to assess the growth and development of children from birth to 5 years of age. These standards are based on primary data collected through the Multicentre Growth Reference Study (MGRS). The MGRS was a population study conducted between 1997 and 2003 in Brazil, Ghana, India, Norway, Oman, and the USA. UU The study combined a longitudinal follow-up from birth to 24 months with a cross-sectional component of children aged 18–71 months. The WHO Child Growth Standards (WHO Standards) adopt a fundamentally prescriptive approach designed to describe how children up to age 5 should grow regardless of their genetic inheritance and where they are born.

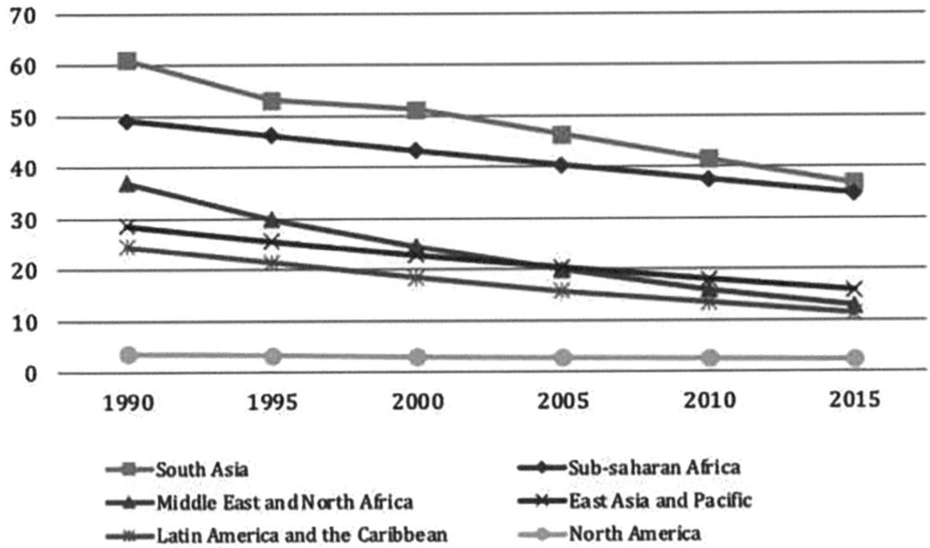

Figure 2.
Child chronic undernutrition rate worldwide by region. Source: UNICEF [8].

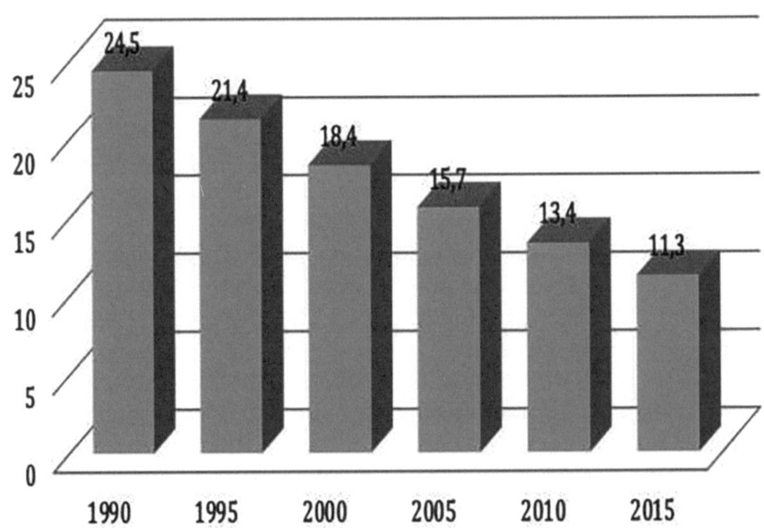

Figure 3.
Child chronic undernutrition rate in Latin America and the Caribbean. Source: with data from UNICEF [8].

year 2015 it was reduced to 11.3%, with this, the prevalence of the region is less than half of the world average (**Figure 3**).

However, this continues to be a public problem in several countries, as there are still around 6 million children under 5 years of age with stunted growth. This indicator would be a reflection of social inequalities in the most unequal region of the planet ([9], p. 5).

Taking into account the heterogeneity of the region, the prevalence by sub-regions was analyzed. Central America has a higher prevalence, reaching about 16%, although its rate of variation on average is higher during the period analyzed, it is

DOI: http://dx.doi.org/10.5772/intechopen.104896

	Caribbean		Central America		South America		Latin America and the Caribbean	
	CCU prevalence	Variation rate per year	CCU prevalence	Variation rate per year	CCU prevalence	Variation rate per year	CCU prevalence	Variation rate per year
1990	16.20		34.10		21.20		24.50	
2000	10.50	0.57	25.70	0.84	16.00	0.52	18.40	0.61
2010	6.60	0.39	18.70	0.70	11.80	0.42	13.40	0.50
2015	5.20	0.28	15.90	0.56	10.10	0.34	11.30	0.42

Source: [11].

Table 1.
Chronic malnutrition rate by subregion in Latin America and the Caribbean [10].

	GDP per cápita	DCI prevalence										
	2015	2005	2006	2007	2008	2009	2010	2011	2012	2013	2014	2015
Brasil	8.757			7.1								
Surinam	8.725						8.8					
China	8.069									8.1		
Nauru	8.053			24								
Gabón	7.389								17.5			
Botsuana	6.532		31.0									
Montenegro	6.514									9.4		
Rep. Dominicana	6.468									7.1		
Turkmenistán	6.433											11.5
Ecuador	6.150										**24.0**	
Colombia	6.045						12.7					
Perú	6.030											14.4
Bielorrusia	5.949	5.0										
Tailandia	5.815								16.3			
Sudáfrica	5.744								27.2			
Azerbaiyán	5.500									18.0		
Serbia	5.237										6.0	
Iraq	4.974							22.6				
Jamaica	4.940										6.2	
Irán	4.862							6.8				

Source: World Bank data (2018).

Table 2.
Latest available CCU prevalence for all countries with GDP per capita is similar to Ecuador.

followed by South America with 10%, and the Caribbean with 5.2%, as can be seen in the following table (**Table 1**).

In turn, within the subregions, there is heterogeneity in the prevalence of chronic child undernutrition between countries. On one hand, there are countries such as Chile (2%) and Costa Rica (6%) with low prevalence, where undernutrition is not pondered as a public problem, and other countries such as Guatemala (49%) and Ecuador (24%) where the prevalence is more than twice that of the region ([12], p. 111; [1], pp. 126–130; [13], p. 15).

By 2015, Ecuador showed a CCU prevalence far from those countries with a similar GDP per capita (**Table 2**).

Although the prevalence of 24% places Ecuador on a similar trajectory to that followed by the indicator worldwide, the phenomenon that motivates this research is that the speed at which the CCU had been reducing until 2004 has slowed down precisely in a period of economic growth.

3. Review of the literature and theoretical framework of the research

The literature on undernutrition, especially that oriented to policy recommendations, usually follows an explanatory scheme of infant undernutrition that identifies three levels in the analysis of the causality of the CCU: immediate causes in the child's organism (or micro), underlying causes at the household level (or meso) and basic causes at the socio-economic (or macro) level (**Figure 4**).

Since the mid-twentieth century, studies on child undernutrition have identified it as a cause and, at the same time, as an effect of poverty: that is, while its immediate manifestations are caused by deprivations associated with poverty, the effects of the undernutrition in the long term seem to perpetuate a condition of poverty. Now, following a chronological order at the individual level, it is accepted that the CCU is a result of poverty or of the conditions of deprivation in the household in which the first

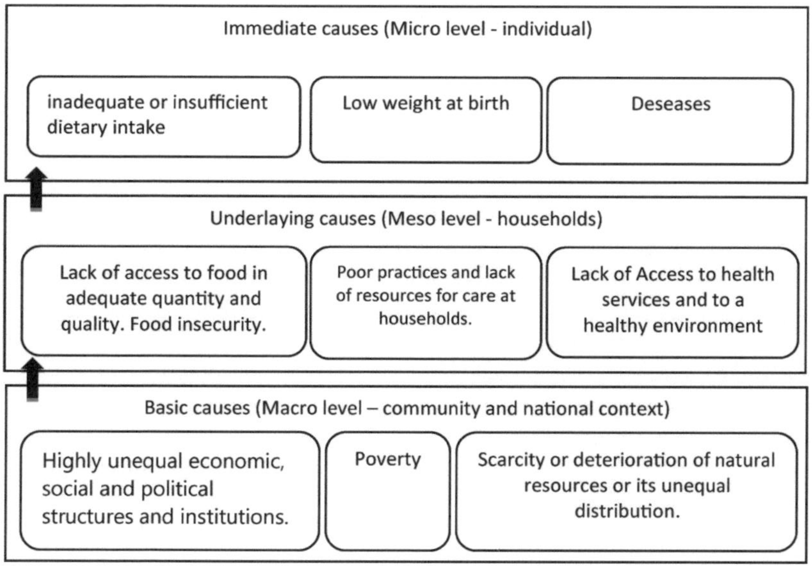

Figure 4.
The causal theoretical model of undernutrition. Source: adapted from UNICEF [16, 17] and from [18].

years of life are developed. It follows that economic growth and its distribution in the segments with the lowest incomes have the potential to reduce the incidence of CCU.

There is abundant evidence on the relationship between nutritional outcomes and income [2, 9, 14, 15]. "It has also been observed that the countries with the greatest reductions in poverty and/or indigence rates have shown the greatest reductions in the CCU rate," whether or not they have programs aimed at improving the growth of boys and girls [14]. According to Headey and others [15] a key factor to explain the sustained nutritional change is the "general economic progress," because it allows more funds to be allocated for food consumption, health, and other items relevant to the nutritional status of the members of the family, especially those younger. However, there are also cases in countries where, even with low economic growth, they have been able to reduce the CCU. Bangladesh is one of these cases, according to the study by Headey and others, the factors that influenced this result were related to the expansion of the economic sectors in which the less favored classes participate (agriculture and manufacturing), they also identified as an effective factor (which had an effect on the problem) the rapid expansion of education since the 1990s, when a policy of subsidies to secondary education was initiated, especially education for women, in fact for 2011 the Demographic and Health Survey (DHS, 2016) found that among mothers and fathers under 25 years of age, mothers had on average one year more education than fathers ([11] in [15]). The authors also considered the development of sanitation infrastructure within their explanatory model. The proportion of villages without sanitation services has decreased from 25.2% in 1997 to 4.8% in 2011. However, improvements in sanitation in Bangladesh have been implemented from a CLTS (Community-led Total Sanitation) approach. It focuses on the change of behavior and not only on large investments in infrastructure. Behavior change, through education, takes more time and requires sustained policies in the long term, this means policies that continue beyond the agendas of governments in office. If these are factors that explain the reduction of the CCU in contexts of low growth or zero growth, then what would be the factors that explain the slowing in the reduction CCU in a context of growth?

While, there has been an inverse correlation between the prevalence of the CCU and economic growth, that is, greater economic growth lower prevalence of the CCU, this correlation is neither clear nor automatic. In this regard FAO has concluded that:

> *There are several key elements in the process that link economic growth, [... and] GDP per capita, with the reduction of undernourishment and undernutrition. First, economic growth must extend to people with a high level of poverty. To reduce poverty and hunger, growth must generate demand for goods controlled by the poor. Second, poor households must use part of the increase in their income to improve their intake of food energy, and other nutrients, as well as to make private investments in health, sanitization facilities, and education. The participation of women is essential to carry out these spending models. Third, a large part of the additional public revenues generated by economic growth should be used to make public sector investments in social protection systems or safety, nutrition, health, and education networks in order to increase the human capital of the poor [...] invest in public goods and services that promote growth in the sectors where the poor work, such as the agriculture sector [...] To ensure the effectiveness and sustainability of these three key elements, good governance at the national level is also fundamental ([11], p. 21).*

A hypothesis derived from this conclusion would be then: economic growth does not translate into improvements in the nutritional status of the child population if such growth does not generate demand for goods controlled by the poor, in other words, when growth does not generate income opportunities for families with less resources. The slowing of the indicator of the CCU could also be related to the practices and habits of consumption of the households, by not allocating the increase in their income to improve the quality of their diet, their state of health, or their sanitary conditions. The persistence of the CCU in growth contexts could also be a result of the lack of investment by governments in social protection systems, in direct measures on nutrition, health, and education of the population.

Thus, understanding why the rate of reduction of the CCU is dormant in a period of economic growth, is a complex task, on the one hand, the explanatory factors could be associated with changes in the variables of the causal model (**Figure 4**) or could be associated to specific conditions of the growth context (derived hypothesis). The factors with the greatest explanatory potential would be those that (i) being part of the causal model of the CCU, (ii) show significant variations in the period analyzed with respect to the previous one and that in turn (iii) are part of the derived hypothesis.

3.1 The causes of CCU in studies on undernutrition in Ecuador

The first national study on the nutritional status of the Ecuadorian population dates from 1959. This determined three central problems: protein-energy undernutrition, that is, the population did not consume the proteins and calories considered necessary for adequate nutrition, endemic goiter, and anemia. Subsequent studies, of lesser scope, focused on determining the prevalence of chronic, acute undernutrition and anemia, in different population groups. In 1988 the Diagnosis of the Nutritional Food Situation of the Ecuadorian Population (DANS) was published. This study had a national scope and constituted a starting point for contemporary analyzes on undernutrition in Ecuador.

The DANS identified the areas of greatest territorial concentration of the CCU and included three types of variables as part of the explanatory model of nutritional status: the social insertion of the head of household (income, occupation, schooling), the degree of risk of housing (overcrowding, water supply, sanitation, floor material and location of the kitchen, garbage collection), and data on childhood morbidity acute undernutrition (diarrheal, respiratory, measles and vaccines).

According to the measurement of this study, 49.4% of children under the age of 5 in the country (623,241 children) suffered from chronic undernutrition; 37.5% suffered from global undernutrition, low weight-for-age, or under-weight (473,108 children) and 4% had low weight-for-height or wasting (50,465 children). It was found that the problem was greater in the Andean rural areas, in this region the CCU affected the children immediately after birth (30% in children from 0 to 6) and it increased to more than double among the 48 and 60 months involving an incidence of undernutrition "from the mother's womb." Likewise, when analyzing the prevalence of CCU in relation to "social insertion," it is noted that "nutritional problems affect socially and economically depressed population groups that do not have access to an income that allows them to satisfy their basic needs," among these, the purchase of food, the availability of basic services and adequate housing conditions. Hence, the study concludes that "the food and nutritional problem is only one of the characteristics of the condition of poverty" ([19], p. 13). Since then, the phenomenon of undernutrition has been identified in rural areas and with populations categorized as poor.

The DANS also concluded that "the housing risk indicator" has a "highly significant" relationship with undernutrition as well as the level of education of the mother, implying that "an improvement in the level of education of the mother would significantly influence the nutritional status of the child." The study mentions that the reduction of chronic undernutrition "requires long and medium-term interventions ... that permanently and substantially modify the living conditions" of the population, as demonstrated by the experience of other countries [19].

Regarding the consumption of food, the study showed that on average and nationally, the children of that time consumed 15.5 g of protein of animal origin, which added to vegetable proteins (15.0 g), indicating protein sufficiency. However, a protein-energy deficiency was observed in the scattered areas of the Sierra and the Coast, in contrast to the urban areas where a caloric deficiency accompanied by a protein surplus appears.

From 1987 until 2004, the Center for Population and Social Development Studies (Cepar) carried out the Demographic and Maternal and Child Health Survey (Endemain). The Endemain of 2004 was a study with national, urban, and rural representation, by regions and provinces, this study found that, at the national level, 23.2% of children under 5 years of age suffered from chronic undernutrition,[3] and within this group, 5.9% had "severe chronic undernutrition" that is, they presented an even greater delay in growth. In the rural area, undernutrition was 30.7%. The indicator in the Sierra (32%), was almost 10 points more than in the Amazon (22.7%) and double that in the coast (15.7%). The Endemain analyzed the distribution of the incidence of the CCU by cities and found that in Quito it was higher (30.2%) than in any other urban area of the Sierra (19.3%). In Tungurahua, Bolívar, Cañar, and Chimborazo, more than 40% of children under the age of five had chronic undernutrition. The CCU increased its incidence from 12 months of age and was higher in children with low weight and short stature at birth, children whose birth had occurred up to 47 months after the previous delivery had a prevalence of 28%, and as the order increased from birth the probability of suffering from CCU increased, for example in the group of firstborn children, the prevalence was 19% while in those who were born seventh or more the prevalence was 41%.

This survey incorporated a component that collected perceptions about food security. It was determined that 16% of the households interviewed stated that they had difficulties feeding their members, in a greater percentage of rural households, among these, the coast region households expressed greater insufficiency than those in the Andes. It was also found that 28% of households had difficulty paying food expenses, in rural households this problem is exacerbated. The strategy to solve the difficulties of access to food is to lend products from the neighborhood stores (66%), this custom is widespread in all regions especially in the Amazon (81%) and in rural households (71%) Another measure is to stop buying some products (64%) and borrow money from family and friends (62%) (these categories are not exclusive). In view of the difficulties of access, 40% of the households surveyed would have resorted to both credit in stores and to suppress the variety of products they consumed. The Endemain 2004, presented descriptive statistical information, of quantitative and categorical variables on the CCU, but does not elaborate on causal models with this information.

Later, in 2007, the World Bank commissioned the elaboration of a profile of the CCU of Ecuador. This study states that in 1986 (using the DANS data and the new [7] tables) the prevalence of CCU was 34%; using the data from the Survey of Living Conditions (SLC) of 1998, a prevalence of 26.4% was calculated, and; using data from the Endemain 2004 [20], a 23.1% prevalence rate was calculated for that year; with these data it was calculated that an annual reduction of six tenths (0.6) had occurred from 1986 to 2004.

[3] These prevalences are calculated with the 1970 reference curves, while the prevalences of the table drawn up by Fernando Carrasco are calculated, using the same database but based on the WHO 2006 curves.

That study uses a method of multivariate regression analysis, that is, to establish the contribution of different factors (independent variables = following the theoretical causal model) to the CCU indicator (Z score or standard deviation from normal value of height-for-age). This model focused on risk factors or more significant factors at the household level: the size of the home, the number of women over 14 years in the home, age, stature, and the expectation of the mother regarding the stature of their children. It was identified as determinant condition of the resources available for the household (measured by per capita and assets), although it is said that this is the "long road" to change and that "other more direct strategies are required to improve nutritional conditions" ([21], p. 30). At the community level (the macro-level factors), it was determined that children in rural areas and in areas of higher altitude, have lower probabilities of growing than those in urban areas and low-lying areas. And that "likely that investment in improving rural sanitation provides positive benefits in nutritional status" ([21], p. 31).

To avoid problems of endogeneity, the model did not include variables related to the behaviors that affect nutritional outcomes. But in additional analysis, they found that breastfeeding, pre and postnatal care, attention during childbirth, and birth control, all impact the nutritional outcomes of children.

When analyzing the data on food consumption, the study concluded that the CCU is related to "the lack of capacity to buy food" and that the main difference in food consumption between households with children with low height for age and children with adequate height is the "percentage of participation of meat in total consumption," which in the second group is higher ([21], pp. 50–64).

In summary, since 1986, several studies have provided increasingly refined explanations about the causes of CCU. Among the immediate or individual-level factors causally related to CCU are low weight at birth, presence of diseases, and birth order. Among the underlying causes are age, height and education of the mother, the mother's expectation regarding the height of her child, breastfeeding practices, the socioeconomic status of the household, the size of the household, the number of children under 5 years of age and women over 14 in the home, the conditions and building materials of the house, per capita food consumption, diet composition, access to health services, access to safe drinking water, and availability of sewage. Among the basic factors are economic inequality, segregation by area, isolation by altitude, ethnic discrimination, poverty, relative prices, and economic shocks ([21], p. 16; [21], pp. 27–39; [22], pp. 217–22; [23], pp. 1–10; [24], p. 361; [25], pp. 3–6).

Finally, in contrast to these studies, this research does not seek to explain the causes of the CCU but is focused on exploring the factors contributing to the slowdown of the CCU prevalence reduction in Ecuador during a period of economic growth. The methodology followed is explained below.

4. Method, data collection and analysis

A mixed, explanatory and sequential method was designed in four phases (**Figure 5**).

Since the objective of this research was to explain the slowdown in the reduction of chronic child undernutrition in the period 2004–2014, indicators were identified for the factors that, according to the multilevel causal model and the studies carried out in the country on the CCU, appear more related to the prevalence in 2004. These values are compared with the same indicators for 2014 to identify changes and continuities. However, since some of these variables have effects in the medium and long term, it was

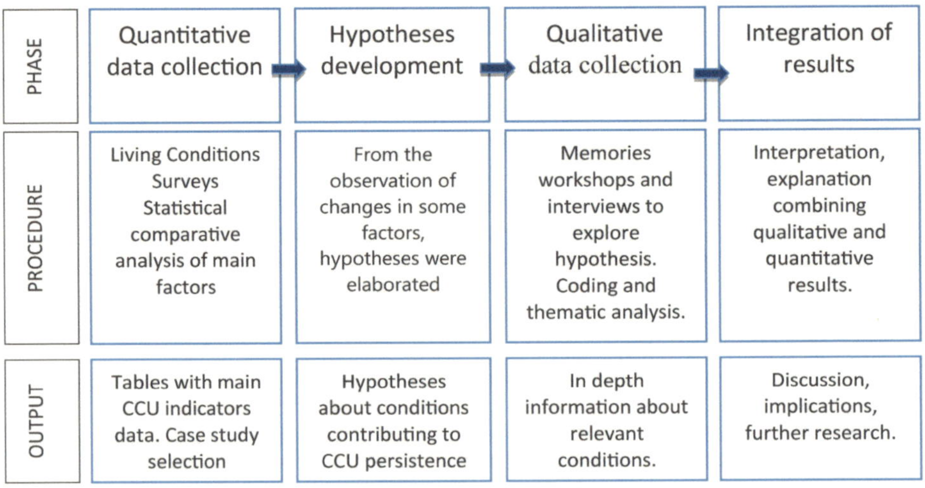

Figure 5.
Sequential explanatory design. Adapted from ([26], p. 39).

necessary to move the analysis back to the previous period for which there is available data on the same indicators. In this case, the Life Conditions Surveys of 1998, 2006, and 2014 were used. Descriptive statistics analysis was carried out for the comparison of indicators, no predictive models or regressions were elaborated since the explanation lies in the observation of variations in the relevant indicators from one period to another. Once the factors that experienced the greatest changes between 2004 and 2014 were identified. In base, to these changes, some hypotheses were constructed. These hypotheses were explored by qualitative inquiry techniques. The qualitative component provided more specific information about the variables identified as relevant in the model and about new variables with explanatory potential. The data were analyzed and interpreted and thus the hypothesis that constitutes the main conclusion of this study was constructed.

A mixed-method was chosen because, often, quantitative causal studies identify the variables that are significantly (positively or negatively) related to the occurrence of a phenomenon but do not offer an explanation of how they occur. These cause-effect relationships in a given context do not allow identifying other factors than those included in the model. Qualitative research helped to obtain a more comprehensive view of the phenomenon by illustrating how certain conditions (macro, meso, and micro) are combined to obtain a result, as well as adding emerging factors observed during the investigation and not included in the theoretical model. The combination (or triangulation) of methods and techniques is considered a necessary research strategy for the field of social sciences, because on the one hand, it allows the study to be provided with a more complete, deep, and broad contextual sense, thus increasing its internal validity, At the same time, the twofold sources of data allow to build conditions for generalization and therefore to extend its external validity ([27], pp. 538–539).

5. Results

In Ecuador, there are measurements of the prevalence of CCU from the 1986 DANS Survey, and the last one can be obtained from the 2014 ECV. Due to the change in the standards of the growth curves, the update of prevalence figures prior to 2006 has generated certain confusion and a lack of continuity in the analysis of trends. Since serial measurements are not available from the same source, to make the figures comparable, it is necessary to make sure that all the data are calculated based on the same parameter and follow the same calculation methodology. In order to have comparable historical indicators of prevalence, for this research, data from different sources were recalculated in different years, using the [7] standard as the only reference parameter, as can be seen in the following table (**Table 3**).

It can be seen that for the period 1986–2014, the CCU has been reduced by 17.1 points, that is, on average, 6 tenths (0.61) per year. However, the trend of this reduction over the years has not been uniform, as shown in the following figure (**Figure 6**).

The slope of the curve clearly shows two periods: the first between 1986 and 2004 in which the rate of reduction was close to 0.83 per year, if this trend had been maintained, the CCU in 2014 would have presented a prevalence of 17, 8%. But as of 2004, a point of inflection is observed in which the CCU is reduced by an average of only 2 tenths per year, that is, 2.1 points in 10 years.

Curiously, these years (2004–2014) correspond to a period of economic growth for Ecuador. As of 2004, the country went through a period of economic recovery, going from a GDP of about 36.5 billion to one of 100 billion dollars in 2014, with a GDP per capita of USD 6273 [34], this classifies it as a medium-high income country according to the parameters used by the World Bank. The annual growth rate has been 4.8% on average during that decade. For years with a GDP of less than 3000 USD, the reduction in the CCU is more prominent than for years in the GDP per capita is higher, in later years the reduction of the CCU becomes almost imperceptible.

Anchored to this growth, public sector spending and investment increased considerably, from 21% in 2006 to almost 35% of GDP in 2014 [35]. Recall that in the derived hypothesis, a necessary condition for growth to translate into improvements in the nutritional status of the population is for the State to invest "in social protection systems or safety, nutrition, health, and education networks in order to increase the human capital of the poor." "During the analyzed period, more than 50% of the total social spending was allocated to the education sector" (around 5% of GDP); to the health sector was allocated the 25%, and the rest in social protection programs [28, 29, 35].

In his analysis of social spending in Ecuador for the period 2006–2012, Naranjo has noticed that although there were adjustments in the parameters of operation of

Years	1986	1998	1999	2000	2004	2006	2014
Chronic childhood undernutrition prevalence	41.1%	32.7%	32.2%	31.0%	26.1%	26.1%	24%
		0.7	0.5	1.2	1.22	0	0.26
Annual variation rates averages			0.71			0.21	
			0.83				
			1.1			0.26	
				0.54			
				0.61			

Sources: DANS-CONADE [19] imputed values: INEC-ECV [28–31]. Employment Survey: INEC-SIEH-ENEMDU [32]. Elaboration: Fernando Carrasco [33].

Table 3.
Chronic childhood undernutrition prevalence in Ecuador 1986–2014.

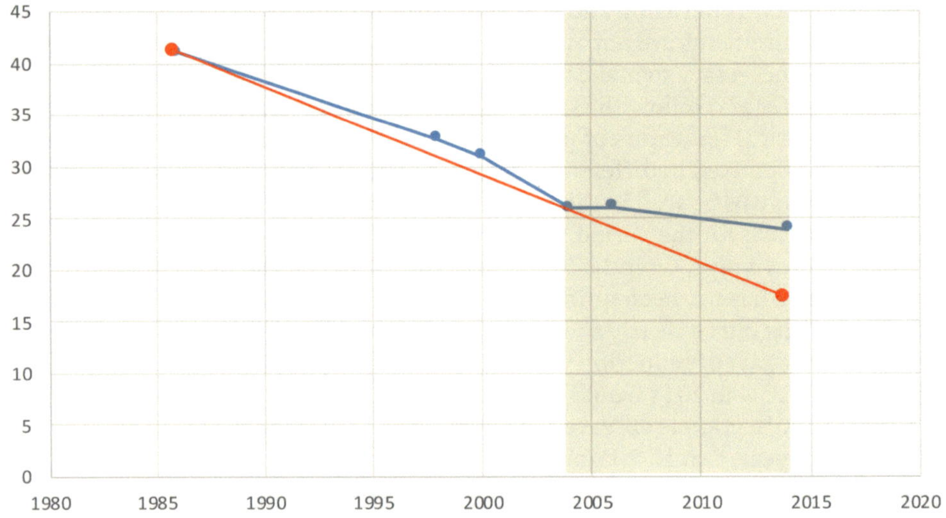

Figure 6.
Chronic childhood undernutrition reduction rate average 1986–2014.

social policies as an increase in the amounts of benefits, in the coverage of care, and improvement In the infrastructures and equipment of social services, there was still no evidence of "structural changes" in social programs. Certainly, a large amount of resources was allocated to investments related to social policy, however, Naranjo questions whether these resources come from non-permanent sources of public income, therefore future financing and the sustainability of the changes were unclear ([36], pp. 77–78).

In the derived hypothesis, it is stated that for economic growth to favor adequate access to food both in quantity (food energy) and in quality (diversity, nutrient content, and safety); this growth would have to include the poor, that is, generate employment and demand for the goods produced by the poor.

In a study conducted in 2011, Ponce found that the growth experienced since 2001 would have been a "pro-poor growth," meaning that "the growth levels of the poorest deciles (were) greater than the growth levels of the richest deciles", unlike the type of growth that was observed for the decade of the 1990s-concentrated in the segments with the highest income [37].

Indeed, between 2004 and 2014, the indicator of poverty by income showed a reduction of fifteen points, going from 44.6 to 22.5%. Since the beginning of the new century, while the per capita GDP and poverty growth indicators show an inverse relationship with simila slopes, the prevalence of CCU remains almost constant (**Figure** 7).

A study by the National Institute for Statistics and Census [39] ensured that, from 2006, the main factor behind the reduction of poverty by consumption was the increase in the income of the quintiles with fewer resources, by way of labor income, as can be seen below (**Table 4**).

Regarding socioeconomic mobility, the study indicates that, despite the fact that there is a high level of persistence, of 100% of the poor in 2006, 41% moved towards vulnerability or middle class. Specifically, 26% of people who were categorized as poor in 2006, became "vulnerable" in 2014 and 15% came to be considered "middle

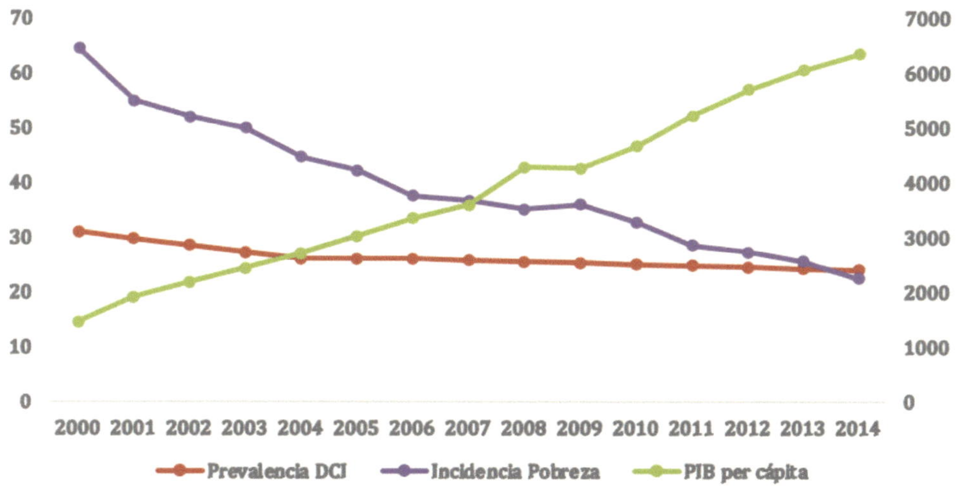

Figure 7.
Trends in GDP, per capita, poverty, and prevalence of the CCU. Source: [38].

	Year	Labor income	Variation %	Total income	Variation %
Total	2006	239.8		323.8	
	2014	298.7	24.6	415.7	28.4
Quintile 1	2006	76.6		94.1	
	2014	107.9	40.9	136.0	44.5
Quintile 2	2006	108.2		134.7	
	2014	163.2	50.8	202.5	50.3
Quintile 3	2006	148.0		206.2	
	2014	207.3	40.1	269.7	30.8
Quintile 4	2006	215.9		289.9	
	2014	275.5	27.6	401.3	38.4
Quintile 5	2006	507.4		694.2	
	2014	569.4	12.2	818.2	17.9

Source and elaboration: INEC SLC, [39], p. 217.

Table 4.
Increase in labor income by quintiles 2006–2014.

class." Of 100% of the population recognized as "vulnerable" in 2006, 27% became middle class.[4] During this period, poverty reduction has been explained, in part (43%), by the real growth of household consumption ([39], p. 21). This growth in turn would be explained by greater access to employment, which for the lowest income quintiles in this period shifted "towards jobs in the sectors of greater value in

[4] Although it was also found that from 100% of vulnerable people in 2006, 7% became poor in 2014, and of the 100% of the middle-class population, 7% became poor and 12% became poor. vulnerable "(INEC, 2016, p. 30).

the economy, particularly trade and construction in urban areas, and agro-export in rural areas" [40].[5]

Although productive activity grew in general, the services sector had the highest growth: 55.4% of GDP. The sectors in which the population with fewer resources works, grew in a smaller proportion: agriculture grew by 6.5% and manufacturing by 11% [41]. Agriculture was the least dynamic sector of the economy during this period between 2007 and 2014, 253,281 jobs were lost. The crops destined for export (banana, coffee, cocoa and flowers, aquaculture and shrimp fishing and forestry) were the ones that contributed most to the growth of the sector. Peasant family agriculture was not a priority in the public policies of this period ([42], pp. 25–26).

It would seem that the situation of people categorized as poor changed during the period of analysis when increasing their income, this allowed them to move towards the higher segments. These changes leave doubts about the type of participation of the poor in growth because although the social policies oriented to these segments improved their infrastructure and coverage (e.g., monetary transfers, public health services and education, etc.) there is no evidence of significant growth in the sectors of the economy in which the less favored sectors participate.

When analyzing the effects of the social policies of the so-called "post-neoliberal" governments in Latin America, Perez-Sainz (2018) found that, in general, these advanced in redistributive terms, by increasing the benefits financed by taxes, generating a package of basic social rights, but less progress was made in generating sufficient formal employment for the poorest and in opening opportunities for the accumulation of small owners, that is, there were no significant advances in the distributive sphere of the means of production ([43], p. 69). According to official figures, 57% of the reduction in poverty during this period would be explained by the "redistribution effect" ([39], p. 21).

6. Comparison of relevant variables

The relevant variables were identified according to the causal theoretical model and the previous studies on the CCU in Ecuador. The behavior of these variables was compared between the group of children with a low height for age and the group of children with the expected height for age. Due to the information available, not all the variables could be operationalized in indicators for the different periods. After overcoming several difficulties to homogenize the information and make it comparative, the following variables were selected (**Table 5**).

7. Data analysis

For the next group of variables, it was possible to make comparisons between the group of children with CCU and children without CCU and within each group.

[5] Hunger and malnutrition have usually been explained as problems of food availability (food stocks according to global production and market dynamics) and/or access. The access can be physical or economic. Physical access is associated with availability while economic access depends on the purchasing power of the household and the level of food prices that could depend, in turn, on physical access (Thomson and Metz, 1998). A household's ability to spend on food is often considered a good indicator of home access (Babu and Sanyal, 2009, p. 9).

Analysis level	Variable	Indicator
Micro: individual, Immediate causes	Weight at birth	Low weight (< 2.5 kg) Normal weight (> 2.5 Kg)
	Presence of diseases	Flu Diarrhea
Meso: Household, Underlying causes	Food access in quantity and quality	Food intake Diet composition
	Household structure and practices	Person in charge of childcare Average number of family members Mother's education. Average years of schooling Health checkups
	Access to water and sanitation facilities	Type of water supply Toilet availability
Macro: Community/Basic causes.	Availability of resources	Consumption poverty Income poverty
	Basic and health services	Water supply coverage Sewerage
	Employment	Type of employment (formal/informal) of mother and father

Table 5.
Definition of variables and indicators.

Surveys of Living Conditions (SLC) were the source for those three years 1999, 2006, and 2014, which include measures of childhood stunting (**Table 6**).

By comparing these data it is possible to conclude the following:

For the group with CCU, the frequency of children with low birth weight increases by 0.9 points for the year 2014 in relation to the previous periods, for the group without CCU this indicator worsens by 2.1 percentage points between 1999 and 2006 It would seem that the presence of this factor has worsened for the group without CCU during the period analyzed.

The presence of diseases such as diarrhea and influenza decreases significantly between 2006 and 2014, both for the CCU group and for the other group, so this individual or micro-level factor could not be identified as a causal variable associated with the slowdown in the decrease of the CCU. The same could be said of the frequency with which children attend routine health checkups, as an indicator of access to health services, this indicator improves a lot for the period between 1999 and 2006, especially for the group with CCU. Therefore, it could not be identified as a causal variable associated with the slowdown in the reduction of the CCU.

With respect to the persons in charge of caring for children, the frequency between the options remains stable in the three moments analyzed and in the two observation groups, except for the last option in which, the group with CCU increases the frequency with which children attend a children's center, while for 1999 only 3.2% of children with IND went to a childcare center, for 2006 this frequency rises to 8, 1% and remains stable until 2014 (7.8%).

The way in which the homes of children with CCU are supplied with water seems to have improved substantially between 2006 and 2014, since 67.2% receive water from the public network, almost 20 points more than in 1999 (**Table 7**).

	Families/Children with CCU			Families/Children without CCU		
Indicator	**1999**	**2006**	**2014**	**1999**	**2006**	**2014**
Low weight (<2.5 kg)	11.7%	11.5%	12.6%	3.9%	6.0%	6.5%
Normal weight (< 2.5 kg)	88.3%	88.5%	87.4%	96.1%	94.0%	93.5%
The child had diarrhea last week	30.9%	28.2%	20.6%	24.0%	23.8%	15.9%
The child had flu last week	54.0%	57.0%	46.7%	60.3%	56.0%	46.8%
Health checkups without being sick.	6.2%	19.1%	22.2%	14.5%	21.7%	24.9%
Child caregiver						
Mother	78.6%	75.6%	77.7%	78.8%	77.1%	76.5%
Father/grandfather/uncle	10.0%	12.6%	11.8%	11.7%	14.2%	14.7%
Home member 10 years and more	5.1%	2.0%	1.7%	4.0%	1.7%	1.8%
Home member < de 10 years	1.9%	0.7%	0.2%	0.2%	0.3%	0.1%
Another relatives, neighbors and friends	0.9%	0.5%	0.4%	1.2%	0.8%	1.1%
Domestic worker or babysitter	0.3%	0.5%	0.4%	1.6%	1.8%	1.0%
Daycare center	3.2%	8.1%	7.8%	2.6%	4.1%	4.7%
Type of water supply						
Public supply	47.6%	49.7%	67.2%	67.2%	63.8%	75.7%
Other source by pipes	23.1%	22.6%	13.0%	9.5%	11.0%	7.8%
Delivery truck or tricycle trike	6.8%	5.9%	2.4%	5.3%	6.6%	3.9%
Water well	9.7%	8.2%	8.8%	9.9%	9.3%	7.8%
River, spring or ditch	10.8%	10.1%	5.4%	6.9%	5.6%	3.2%
Another	2.1%	3.5%	3.3%	1.3%	3.8%	1.6%
Consumption poverty						
Poor	79.9%	67.3%	52.4%	56.0%	44.8%	31.8%
Non poor	20.1%	32.7%	47.6%	44.0%	55.2%	68.2%

Source: INEC-SLC [28, 29, 31].

Table 6.
Comparison of indicators.

In general, housing conditions that, since the first studies on the CCU in Ecuador were identified as a causal variable, seem to have improved especially for the population group categorized as poor, the improvement is greater in terms of the supply of water from the public network and to adequate sanitation.

With regard to the poverty-for-consumption variable, it can be seen that for the year 1999, only 21% of the children identified as stunted were within the group identified as "not poor." In 2006, this indicator rose to 32.7% and by 2014 almost half of the children with CCU (46%) belonged to families categorized as "not poor" (**Table 8**).

These data lead us to think that the CCU has stopped becoming a problem of economic access to food, a problem that has been distinctive in social groups having

Variable	2006		2014	
	Poor	Non poor	Poor	Non poor
Overcrowding	47.5	11.5	36.4	7.3
Public supply water	62.6	85.6	72.5	89.5
Proper sanitation	61.5	91.6	76.6	95.0
Suitable flooring material	82.5	96.9	86.6	97.4
Suitable wall material	80.7	94.1	86.9	96.0
Suitable roofing material	94.2	98.1	98.0	99.8

Source: INEC [44], p. 31.

Table 7.
Changes in housing conditions 2006–2014.

Year	Children population < 5 years	Chronic child undernutrition prevalence	Total	Poor	%	Nonpoor	%
1999	1280860	32.20%	412436	325825	79%	86611	21%
2006	1406536	26.10%	367106	245961	67%	121145	33%
2014	1556339	24%	373521	201702	54%	171820	46%

Source: Data of SLC [28, 29, 31] processed by Fernando Carrasco [33] in ***Table 6****.*

Table 8.
Population with CCU according to poverty by consumption.

fewer resources, and that now this problem has permeated the segments of the population with higher income.

8. Territorial distribution of the CCU

In order to advance in the definition of specific territories for qualitative research, the distribution of prevalence's by provinces was analyzed, since this is the level at which the SLC allows the data to be disaggregated. The results were compared and the territories in which the CCU has decreased above and below the national average for the three periods analyzed were identified. These territories were chosen as case studies (**Table 9**).

It is observed that the provinces in which there was a greater reduction of the CCU, between 2006 and 2014, were the provinces identified as critical, for their high prevalence, Cotopaxi and Chimborazo for example, although they still have high prevalence, they decreased 10 and 8 points respectively, Imbabura decreased almost 11 points, in all three cases the biggest change occurred in the rural sector. On the other hand, Carchi, Esmeraldas, and Pichincha raise their prevalence between 5 and 2 points, but when looking at the indicator disaggregated by area of residence, it is observed that in Carchi the prevalence increases 9 points in the urban area while in the rural area it remains constant. On the contrary, in Pichincha, the prevalence increases by 10 points in the rural area and more than two points in the urban area.

Province	Total		Urban		Rural	
	2006	2014	2006	2014	2006	2014
Azuay	37.7	31.5	28.7	24.3	46.9	40.0
Bolívar	47.8	40.1	23.7	22.4	53.2	46.6
Cañar	35.1	30.6	21.1	25.9	44.7	34.6
Carchi	30.4	35.1	25.7	34.7	35.7	35.6
Cotopaxi	43.7	33.7	29.8	25.5	48.0	37.0
Chimborazo	52.8	44.9	31.6	34.1	61.1	49.7
El Oro	15.1	13.7	13.8	13.1	20.2	16.4
Esmeraldas	19.5	21.5	16.7	19.8	22.5	24.3
Guayas	17.4	16.6	14.7	16.0	29.0	20.7
Imbabura	40.8	29.9	30.9	27.1	55.0	35.5
Loja	34.7	27.2	19.7	20.5	42.1	35.1
Los Ríos	22.8	18.5	23.5	17.5	22.0	19.8
Manabí	25.2	19.0	24.5	16.0	26.0	24.1
Morona Santiago		43.6		28.1		48.0
Napo		29.8		13.7		35.5
Pastaza		35.1		21.4		41.7
Pichincha	22.6	26.2	22.1	24.7	25.2	35.7
Tungurahua	35.6	33.1	21.4	21.0	45.4	42.2
Zamora Chinchipe		30.1		21.5		33.8
Galápagos		17.0		19.7		8.3
Sucumbíos		25.4		16.1		30.4
Orellana		26.6		18.2		32.1
Santo Domingo de los Tsachilas		16.2		15.4		19.9
Santa Elena		40.2		39.4		47.1

Source: SLC [28, 29, 31]. Elaboration: Fernando Carrasco [33].

Table 9.
Prevalence of the CCU by provinces of Ecuador.

In Esmeraldas and Guayas prevalence rise in the urban area. While some territories improved radically (Imbabura, Cotopaxi) others worsened (Pichincha) or improved very little (Tungurahua).

With these results, two rural parishes of Pichincha and one in Chimborazo were selected as study cases, where the changes in prevalence are greater.

Surveys that collect information on household spending patterns with a focus on food, calorie consumption, consumption of major products, and socioeconomic characteristics are useful for assessing access to food over time, estimating quantities of food consumed, the composition of the diet, and the availability of nutrients at the individual and household levels ([45], p. 9).

With the information from the National Survey of Income and Expenses of the Ecuadorian Households—ENIGHUR, the consumption of food of the households for the years 2003–2004 and 2011–2012 was analyzed since this information is available only for those two periods. The foods are grouped by class. Consumption is divided

FOOD GROUPS	Total	Quintile 1	Quintile 2	Quintile 3	Quintile 4	Quintile 5
Bread and cereals	16.40%	21.30%	17.90%	15.70%	14.30%	13.90%
Meat	20.50%	18.60%	20.80%	21.00%	20.90%	20.80%
Fish	5.80%	6.20%	5.80%	5.60%	5.60%	5.60%
Milk, Cheese and Eggs	15.30%	12.20%	13.40%	14.40%	16.70%	19.00%
Oil and Fats	3.10%	4.50%	3.80%	2.90%	2.50%	2.10%
Fruits	9.10%	6.20%	7.40%	8.70%	10.10%	12.40%
Legumes—Vegetables	13.10%	13.30%	13.60%	13.50%	13.00%	12.10%
Sugar, jam, honey, chocolate and sugar candies	2.40%	3.30%	2.90%	2.30%	2.00%	1.80%
Non-alcoholic beverages	5.90%	4.90%	5.70%	5.90%	6.20%	6.80%
Coffee, Tea, Cocoa	1.00%	1.30%	1.10%	0.90%	0.90%	0.80%
Mineral Waters Soft Drinks, Fruit and Vegetable Juices	4.90%	3.50%	4.60%	5.00%	5.30%	6.00%
Others non specified	8.40%	9.60%	8.60%	10.00%	8.70%	5.50%

Source: INEC—National Survey of Income and Expenses of Ecuadorian Households—ENIGHU, [46].

Table 10.
Expenditure by monthly household consumption by income quintile (2003–2004).

by quintile. The value corresponds to the percentage of the total expenditure that households allocate to each food group (**Table 10**).

For the 2003–2004 period, it can be observed that the largest share of food expenditure in households categorized in quintile 1 is allocated to bread and cereals, that is, to carbohydrate sources. The second item in participation is the meats, and in third place are the vegetables. For Quintile 2, the relationship between meat and cereals is inverted and the share of non-alcoholic beverages increases, as does the share of mineral waters, soft drinks, and fruit juices. In quintile 5, the share of meat is similar to that of the intermediate quintiles (20.8%), but the participation of bread and cereals is lower, as is the participation of the group of dairy products and eggs. In this quintile, the participation of fruits rises. The share of "sugar, jam, honey, chocolate and sweets" is much lower than the share of the same food group in quintile 1. In this quintile, the share of soft drinks and mineral waters, soft drinks, and fruit juices are greater than in the lower quintiles. The participation of vegetables is similar in all quintiles, although it drops more than one point in quintile 5.

The following analysis is presented for the years 2011–2012 (**Table 11**).

For the years 2011–2012, the participation of bread and cereals in the consumption of all the quintiles increased. In quintile 1 the participation of the meat is slightly reduced. In this quintile and in the 2, the participation of dairy products and eggs decreases, and the participation of the group of oils and fats increases, as does that of sugars and sweets. In quintile 5 the participation of meat and fruit falls, and the

Food groups	Total	Quintile 1	Quintile 2	Quintile 3	Quintile 4	Quintile 5
Bread and cereals	18.80%	24.20%	21.00%	18.60%	17.00%	14.60%
Fresh and frozen meats	19.60%	18.10%	20.00%	20.50%	20.20%	18.90%
Fresh, processed, chilled and frozen fish and shellfish	5.80%	6.40%	5.90%	5.70%	5.70%	5.30%
Milk, derivatives and eggs	14.00%	10.70%	12.70%	14.10%	14.80%	16.70%
Oils and fats	3.60%	5.40%	4.40%	3.50%	2.90%	2.20%
Fruits	9.10%	7.00%	7.80%	8.70%	9.90%	11.70%
Vegetables, greens, legumes and tubers	13.00%	14.00%	13.40%	13.30%	12.90%	11.90%
Sugar, jam, honey, chocolates and sugar candies.	3.60%	4.70%	3.80%	3.30%	3.10%	3.10%
Non-alcoholic beverages	10.40%	7.20%	8.70%	10.20%	11.60%	13.50%
Coffee, tea, cocoa and aromatic herbs	1.10%	1.30%	1.20%	1.00%	1.00%	0.90%
Mineral waters, soft drinks, juices, fruit and vegetable juices	9.40%	5.90%	7.60%	9.10%	10.60%	12.60%
Others non specified	2.10%	2.30%	2.20%	2.10%	2.00%	2.10%

Source: INEC—National Survey of Income and Expenses of Ecuadorian Households—ENIGHU, [47].

Table 11.
Expenditure for monthly household consumption by income quintile (2011–2012).

participation of sweets and sugars, non-alcoholic beverages and mineral waters, soft drinks, and processed fruit juices increases significantly. These last two items went up for all the quintiles.

In summary, there is a growing trend in the participation of bread and cereals (mainly rice), lower consumption of meats, dairy products, and eggs while the consumption of sugars and processed and processed beverages increases.

This analysis shows us the participation of food groups in the diet and, although indirectly, it offers us information about the changes in the consumption of certain food groups, for example, the greater participation of sugars, fats, and processed beverages suggest some elements consider as a hypothesis that consumption habits and practices are moving towards food groups with lower nutritional value.

In order to test this hypothesis, quantitative information was complemented with qualitative research.

8.1 Results of qualitative research

Once the case studies for qualitative research have been identified (San Martín de Porres and Recinto Solaya de Mindo, province of Pichincha, and the San Pablo de Gramapamba community in Chimborazo) as well as the categories on which to deepen the qualitative inquiry (changes in the practices and habits of food consumption in the last decade 2004–2014 with respect to the previous one) a specific methodology was designed to obtain qualitative information. "Memories workshops" (80 people participating) were organized and on-site interviews were conducted (20 people interviewed). The information obtained in all three cases was systematized coded and categorized to identify similarities and differences in food consumption habits and practices.

The most striking finding of the qualitative component was that no radical differences were observed regarding feeding practices and habits between the information collected in cases in which the CCU increased considerably and the case in which the CCU decreased.

Among the main conclusions of qualitative research is the perception that the last decade was a time of modernization. As evidence of this, it is mentioned that the coverage of electricity in households increased and with it the use of electrical appliances, and of communication technologies. It improved the road network and with it increased the physical access to new foods, in addition to the fresh local foods that were traditionally consumed, the neighborhood small stores of the community were supplied with processed products such as yogurts, fried foods, and sweeties. The participation of this type of food increased in the diet, especially among the youngest ones. Even the school breakfast given in the public schools of these communities consists of processed foods.

This change is also observed in the behavior of parents who now have more income that allows them to buy processed foods which they send as lunch for school. This was observed in all the cases analyzed, even in rural areas where families have access to some small agricultural products. The purchase of processed foods is identified as an expression of the new purchasing power of families. Among traditional products, rice is still consumed as the main ingredient for lunch.

Perhaps the perception of a more radical change is observed in the Gramapamba Community, where it is reported that during the 90s and early 2000s, the diet included tubers such as melloco, oca, and mashua; and at least 7 varieties of potatoes, in addition to legumes such as beans (tender and dried) lupine, white corn and green peas; cereals such as quinoa, barley, chilli (variety of barley), rye, maize and wheat; and other native foods such as chimuila, murunga, and Cape gooseberrys. As for meats, the consumption of guinea pig, beef, sheep, goat, pig, chicken, and rabbit was mentioned, they were of generalized consumption.

It is recalled that the preparation of traditional foods was a labor that took a long time and required a lot of work on the part of the women (for example cleaning, roasting, and grinding the barley in stone to do the machica). Foods such as chiguilo (a dish made with potatoes and wrapped with corn leaves), barley rice, llapingachos, and drinks such as chawar mishki (drink extracted from penco) that were part of the ordinary diet are mentioned.

Now young people have stopped using the machica to find it unpleasant to taste compared to other foods of lower nutritional quality. The same happens with dishes made with mashua. These food preferences have affected the production of food in the community. The daily consumption of rice and sweets and fried snacks, cookies, potato chips, and soft-sweetened drinks, especially preferred by children, has increased. These are products that are also available at schools. With regard to newborns, breast milk continues to be the main source of food, and in recent years new foods have been incorporated since the seventh month, according to the recommendations of the health professionals.

The practice of credit in the neighborhood small stores is mentioned when money is not available to buy food. The products available in these pantries are mainly processed foods, since fresh foods are sold in local markets where there is no possibility of credit to buy.

Among the emerging factors with explanatory potential arose internal migration, in the case of Gramapamba, a rural parish of Guamote in Chimborazo, it was estimated that at least one-third of the members of the community have emerged in the last decade to settle definitively or temporarily in other central cities or with more job offers. The Solaya and San Martin de Porres, grounds are rather territories receptors,

Before 2000	**Period 2006–2016**
Breakfast	
For men going to work: Rice, peanut sauce, onion, bread, milk, coffee. For other members of the family: herbal tea with bread, cocoa, sometimes bread with cheese, Green banana with coffee and cheese Machica (barley toasted flour with muscovado) and water. Milk and bread with cheese	Juice, chopped fruit with yogurt, cocoa with bread sometimes with cheese. Oatmeal drink. Muscovado's beverage or black coffee, and bread.
Lunch	
Regular: Noodle soup, legumes soup, locros (thick potato soup), and vegetables soups. Rice with egg and maduro (fried ripe banana), when possible with beef or sausage. Rice with lentils, beans, roasted peanuts, and so on. Second plate: cow, pig and chicken eat, spaghetti, rice, potato, tortillas with salad, cow tripe, yucca with peanuts. meats. On special occasions: first plate: morocho (crushed white corn), chicken leg's broth, barley rice, chuchuca (crushed yellow corn), locros (thick soup of bean, pumpkin, quinoa), cream soups (bean, corn), sancocho (chunky soup with green banana, yuca and meat or fish).	Noodle or green banana soups. Rice with egg, can tuna fish, can sardines. Grains stews, potatoes, legumes. French fries. White corn, and other legumes. Instant soups. Seasoning cubes. Salads: Pea, carrot, corn, beetroot with carrot, tomato, onion, mayonnaise, tomato sauce, and herbs. Other ingredients: beans, onion, garlic, carrot, celery, coriander, noodle, salt rice, and tomatoes On special occasions: chicken, baked or fried pig. Going to a restaurant.
Dinner	
Same as at lunch (two plates, soup and rice with side dishes). Coffee with bread. Fruit or cereal thick beverages (milk with banana, wheat, quinoa, or cereal flour)	Same as at lunch (one plate). Coffee or milk with bread.
Snacks	
Roasted corn Toasted beans Banana with bread Geese with honey—milk Sweet potato Lupine and toasted corn Chapo (machica-barley toasted flour with muscovado and milk or water) Muscovado with cheese.	Processed fruit juices Green fried banana French fries Biscuits Yogurt Milk Bananas

Table 12.
Foods that are part of the diet in the periods selected for the study.

perhaps because of their proximity to centers with greater economic dynamism, the first near the center of Mindo which in recent years experienced a boom in the tourism sector and the second in the borders of the Metropolitan District of Quito, receives immigrant population from other provinces, many come from Chimborazo and Cotopaxi.

Below, is a summary of the foods that were mentioned as part of the diet of the people interviewed for the two periods analyzed (**Table 12**).

In-depth interviews also included perceptions about the role of women in family care, the idea of modernization also appears associated with the emergence of conflicts in gender relations; In recent years, women have more frequently linked to salaried work (formal and non-formal), which would have caused a vacuum of care within the family, the traditional role within the home, assigned to women in patriarchal societies blurs, however, have not changed towards a more equitable redistribution of care tasks between men and women, in several cases, the multiple burdens of tasks for women that should divide their day between family care and work outside the home are evident. Another aspect that was mentioned, repeatedly, was the increase in teenage pregnancies, which in most cases must face alone and without adequate preparation, in the care of their children.

8.2 Quantitative analysis of emerging variables

The variables of internal migration and female employment were analyzed to explore their potential as explanatory factors.

Regarding internal migration, the data on place of birth and place of residence disaggregated by province for the 2010 census are presented below (**Figure 8**).

Provinces identified with major changes in the prevalence of CCU observed that while Pichincha province is the largest population receiver internally, other provinces such as Imbabura, Cotopaxi, Bolivar, and Chimborazo which had significant reductions in the CCU, have traditionally been ejectors. Certainly, this finding is not sufficient to say that the improvement in indicators of CCU in the provinces identified as an ejector, is due to the exodus of its population, however, this is a factor to consider in further inquiries. The immigration toward two central provinces is an indicator of the lack of employment opportunities and social mobility in the provinces of the interior of the country and, even more so, in the rural sector.

Regarding the connection of women to the labor market in recent years, female employment rates for 2007 and 2014 were compared, according to the type of employment (formal/informal) and according to quintiles of the population, obtaining the following results (**Table 13**).

Between 2007 and 2014, more than 390 thousand women joined the labor market, the rate of growth of female employment was higher than the average rate of growth of the population in this period (1.6), therefore this incorporation was important, and it could have an impact on the structure of the families, as well as on the quantity and quality of the care available at the household level. Another relevant issue here is that the largest increase was in the formal labor market, probably due to the employment regulations that were implemented during this period. Regarding the distribution of new jobs by quintile of the population, the data are the following (**Table 14**).

It is observed that for 2014, the segment belonging to quintile 4 increased considerably its share in the female employment distribution, while quintiles 2 and 3 had lower growth rates.

ECUADOR: POPULATION RECEIVING PROVINCES AND POPULATION EXPULSORS
(In thousands)
1990: census

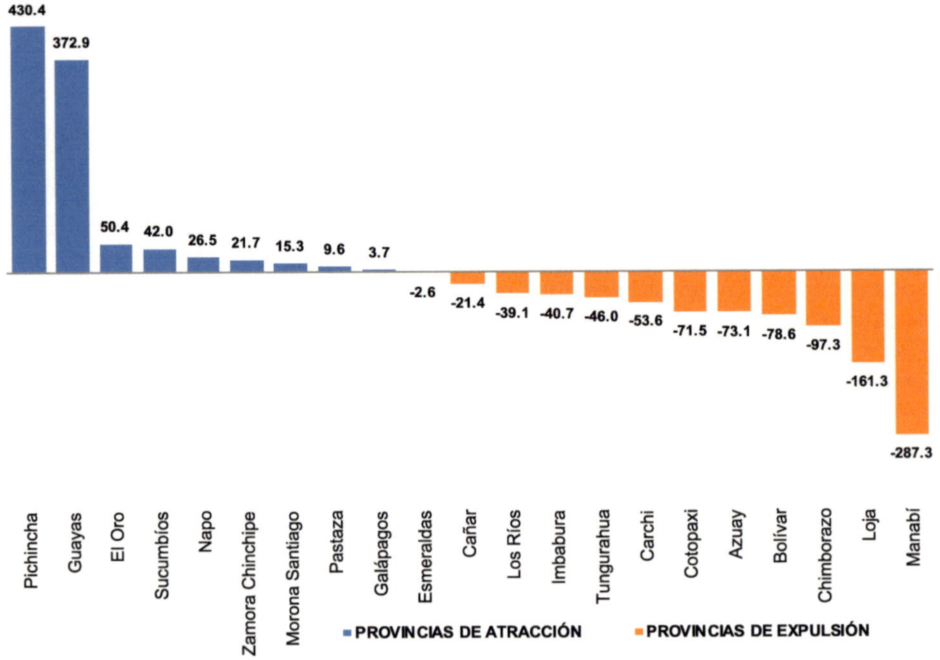

ECUADOR: POPULATION RECEIVING PROVINCES AND POPULATION EXPULSORS
(Per thousands)
2001: census

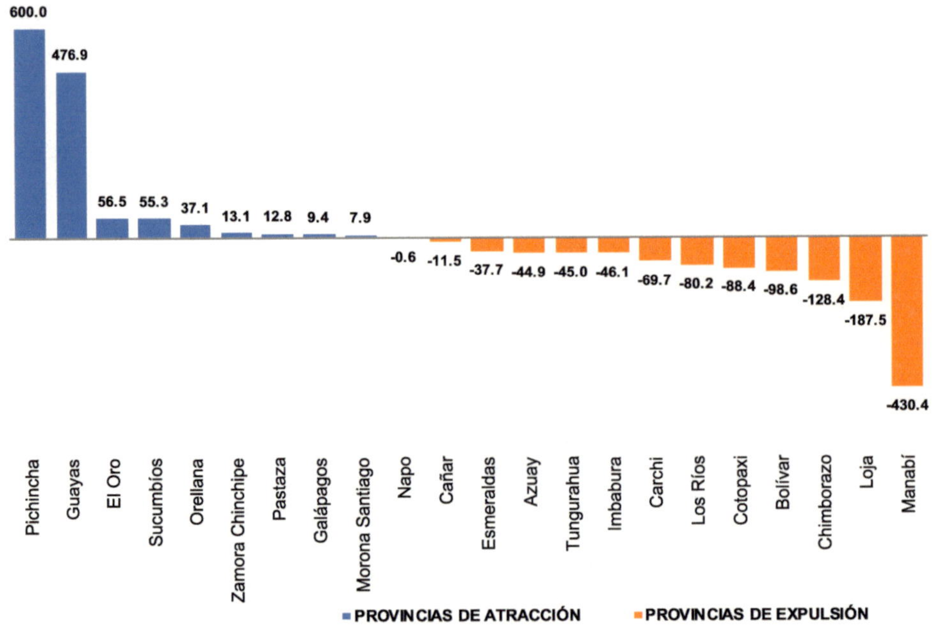

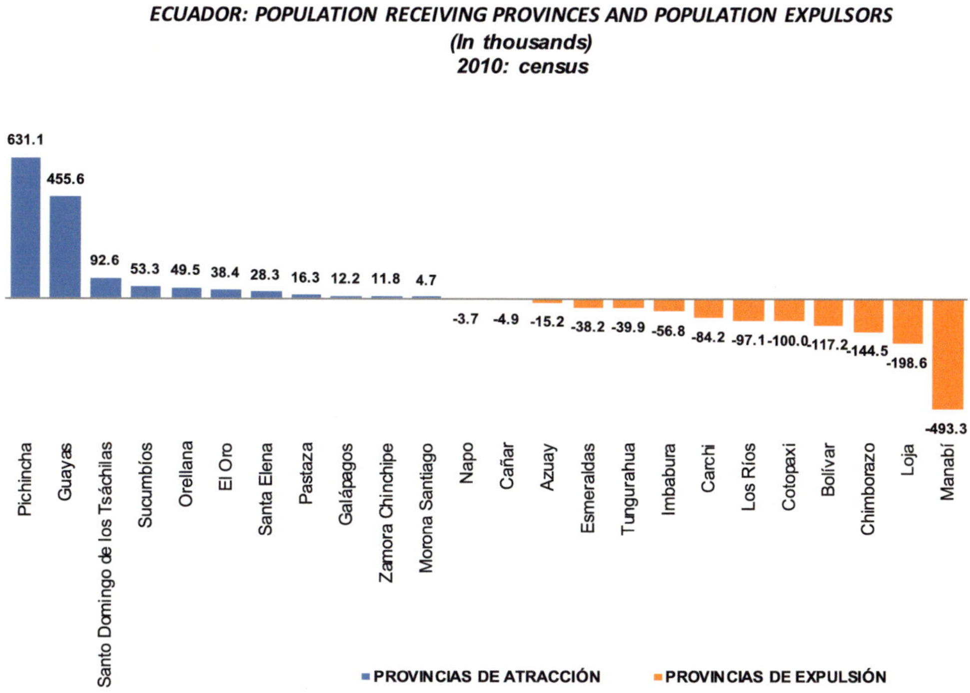

Figure 8.
ECUADOR: Population receiving provinces and population expulsors (in thousands). Source: [48].

Year	Female formal employment		Female Informal employment		NACIONAL	
2007	946 003		1 095 398		2 351 800	
2014	1 317 283	39.2%	1 132 817	3.4%	2 742 189	16.5%
Source: [49].						

Table 13.
Employed female population, by type of employment.

	2007	2014	Difference	%
Quintile 1	419,790	473,871	54,081	13%
Quintile 2	417,382	464,740	47,358	11%
Quintile 3	476,463	530,538	54,075	11%
Quintile 4	513,106	653,442	140,336	27%
Quintile 5	525,058	619,598	94,540	18%
National	2,351,800	2,742,189	390,390	17%
Source: [49].				

Table 14.
Occupied feminine population, per quintiles.

9. Discussion

As we saw in the figures presented at the beginning of this study, Ecuador shows a prevalence of CCU very distant from other countries in the region that had a similar per capita GDP in 2015. Although the prevalence of 24% places the country on a trajectory similar to that followed by the indicator worldwide, the phenomenon that motivated this research was the slowdown in the reduction of the CCU within a context of economic growth between 2004 and 2014.

As the quantitative data collected shows this was a period of socioeconomic mobility in which 41% of the population considered as poor moved to higher strata. 26% stopped being poor and became "vulnerable" and 15% became part of the "middle class." This decrease has been explained both by the growth of household purchasing power via salaries and by redistributive measures from the State. Although there is a generalized growth in employment, including the first quintiles, there is no evidence to suggest that this growth has had a positive impact on the sectors of the economy in which, for the most part, the population with the lowest income, namely small-scale agriculture, which in addition participates in manufacture.

According to the statistics prepared for this study, the tendency of the prevalence of the CCU clearly shows two periods: the first between 1986 and 2004 in which the rate of reduction was about 0.83 per year, and another that goes from 2004 to 2014 in which it is observed a point of inflection in which the CCU is reduced by an average of only 2 tenths per year, that is, 2.1 points in 10 years. This occurs in a period in which GDP per capita rises and poverty decreases.

Many studies have suggested, an inverse correlation between the prevalence of CCU and economic growth, but this correlation is neither direct nor automatic. As we see in the global and national literature review, on the one hand, some of the causal factors of CCU could change its trajectory and influence the prevalence of CCU. On the other hand, and following the FAO literature, it is likely that growth does not translate into improvements in the nutritional status of the child population if such growth does not generate income opportunities for families with fewer resources; if the households do not allocate the increase of their income to improve the quality of their diet, their state of health or their sanitary conditions; and/or if governments do not allocate the fruits of growth to improve their social protection systems, to implement direct measures on nutrition, health and education of the population. These three conditions make up what we have called here a derived hypothesis.

Since there are many possibilities to explain the slowdown, this research selected as factors with greater explanatory potential those that i) forming part of the causal model of the CCU, ii) show significant variations in the period analyzed with respect to the previous one and that its once iii) they are part of the derived hypothesis.

To identify the main causal factors of the CCU in Ecuador, the conclusions of the historical studies were reviewed. The 1988 DANS identified three types of variables as part of the explanatory model: the socioeconomic level of the family, the state of the home, and data on infant morbidity. In the territorial distribution of the problem, was found to be concentrated in rural areas of the Andes. Since that first study, the CCU was identified as a feature of poverty. Later studies included other causal factors; those help us to figure out a causal model. However, the availability of data is a constraint that prevents building an exhaustive model.

Considering a non-exhaustive causal model, the indicators for which there is information available in the SLC of the analyzed period were compared. Thus, at the micro-level, it is observed that the low birth weight and the presence of childhood diseases such as diarrhea and flu do not have significant variations for the different groups analyzed, therefore, these factors do not seem to be related to the slowdown of the CCU. The same applies to the indicator of access to health services.

Regarding the caring indicator, it is observed that the trend follows an expected pattern throughout the period, except that, for the group with CCU, the frequency with which children attend a children's center increases, while In 1999, only 3.2% of children with CCU went to a child care center. In 2006, this frequency rises to 8.1% and remains stable until 2014 (7.8%).

As the figures show, the water supply and the sanitation indicator have substantially improved the analyzed period, which allows for discarding these as factors associated with the slowdown. In general terms, housing conditions seem to have improved especially for the population group categorized as poor.

The data of SLC shows significant variations in the poverty by consumption, given that for the year 1999, only 20% of the children identified with a low height for age, were within the group identified as "not poor," while for 2014 almost half of the children with CCU (47.6%) belonged to this stratum. This allows us to conclude that the CCU is no longer associated with the problems of economic access to food. This significant variation allows us to raise a hypothesis about the slowdown. It is that the CCU has ceased to be a problem of economic access to food and has moved to the upper strata in which the CCU can be explained mainly by the quality of the diet.

Analysis of the territorial distribution shows that the provinces where there was a greater reduction in CCU, between 2006 and 2014, were the provinces historically identified as critical for their high prevalence of CCU: Cotopaxi and Chimborazo decreased by 10 and 8 points respectively, Imbabura decreased almost 11 points, in the three cases the biggest change occurred in the rural sector. In Carchi the prevalence increases by 9 points in the urban area, in Pichincha it rises by 10 points in the rural area. In Esmeraldas and Guayas prevalence rise in the urban area.

To test the second proposition of the derived hypothesis according to which growth translates into improvements in nutritional status if households allocate the increase in their income to improve the quality of their diet, an analysis of the changes in participation was made by food groups in total food consumption, and by quintiles for the years 2003–2004 and 2011–2012, for which there is information available, it is observed that the participation of sources of carbohydrates, sugars and processed beverages increases, as well Protein sources fall, especially in quintile 1 and 2. Indirectly, this information allows us to identify changes in consumption habits and the quality of the diet. To investigate these factors in-depth, qualitative research was carried out. The selection of cases was made based on the findings of the territorial distribution analysis. The qualitative research shows us the perception on the part of the participants about changes in their feeding practices. There is a widespread perception of modernization, change, and economic growth in the last decade. The incorporation into the salaried market even in rural areas has allowed a greater purchasing power for families. But that increase in income goes to buying other processed foods and less fresh, traditional, or natural foods.

Among the emerging categories, the variable of internal migration emerged, from the provinces of the interior to the central provinces where employment opportunities were expanded in recent years. Pichincha, where the CCU increased 10 points in the rural sector, is the main receiving province of the country, while the provinces that have traditionally been critical for the CCU are expellers. However, the data corresponds to the 2010 Census and the level of disaggregation is not sufficient to relate the increase or decrease of the CCU in a territory with the migration of its population.

The second emergent category, the significant connection of women to the labor market in recent years, could have impacted the structure of families, as well as the quantity and quality of care available within households. Although female employment did not grow equitably in all quintiles, it is clear that women in quintiles 1 and 2 contributed to the increase in family income through wages.

Thus, the slowdown in the reduction of the CCU could be explained by the confluence of the following factors: during the period analyzed, many households that until 2006 were identified as poor, became a segment of "vulnerable" or middle-class families, their consumption habits changed, but not necessarily towards an improvement in the nutritional status of the family, the opportunities concentrated in salaried work in certain sectors of the economy, the mobility of the population and the crisis of care could be behind the inconvertibility of new income in better eating habits and feeding practices. In this case, the increase in GDP does not meant, necessarily, different dietary habits for the community in one decade.

This study was exploratory, trying to observe and identify those factors contributing to the slowing down of CCU reduction during an economic growth period in Ecuador, certainly, the study has its own limitations, it would be noteworthy to continue investigating why and how irregular income growth distribution may lead to unexpected results of CCU, and also how and how the background culture of targeted families plays a role guiding the feeding practices in contexts of social and economic change.

Acknowledgements

To carry out this research I had the generous support of Fernando Carrasco, who prepared the database analyzes to determine the prevalence indicators of CCU using the surveys of living conditions. I had the assistance of academic researchers Jairo Rivera and Susana Anda who I was able to work with thanks to the Academic Development Fund (FDA) provided by Flacso-Sede Ecuador. I also received a dedicated support from Sarai García, José Daniel Merchán and Sandra Al Nijjar, scholarship students of the Master's Degree in Public Policy 2018-2020 at Flacso.

Author details

Margarita Manosalvas
Facultad Latinoamericana de Ciencias Sociales, Sede, Ecuador

*Address all correspondence to: mmanosalvas@flacso.edu.ec

References

[1] International Food Policy Research Institute (IFPRI). Global Nutrition Report 2015: Actions and Accountability to Advance Nutrition & Sustainable Development. Washington: IFPRI Institute; 2015

[2] Smith and Haddad. Reducing child undernutrition: Past drivers and priorities for the post-MDG era. In: Revista World Development. Vol. 68. Elsevier Ltd.; 2015. pp. 180-204

[3] Hoddinott J, Alderman H, Behrman JR, Haddad L, Horton S. The economic rationale for investing in stunting reduction. GCC Working Paper Series, GCC. 2013

[4] World Bank. Indicators: GDP per capita Ecuador 1986-2014. 2014. Available from: http://datos.bancomundial.org/indicador/NY.GDP.PCAP.CD [Visit on: 05.15.2014. 14:15]

[5] United Nations Standing Committee on Nutrition. Sixth report on the world nutrition situation. 2010. Retrieved from https://www.unscn.org/files/Publications/RWNS6/report/SCN_report.pdf

[6] Onis M, Garza C, Onyango AW, Martorell R, WHO Multicentre Growth Reference Study Group. Assessment of linear growth differences among populations in the WHO Multicentre Growth Reference Study. Acta Paediatrica. 2006;**450**:56-65

[7] WHO. Training Course on the Evaluation of Child Growth. Version N ° 1. Geneva: World Health Organization; 2006

[8] UNICEF, WHO, & World Bank. Global Overview Child Malnutrition Regional Trends, 1990-2016. 2017. Retrieved June 7 2019, from: http://apps.who.int/gho/data/node.wrapper.nutrition-2016?lang=en

[9] Martínez R, Fernández A. Child undernutrition in Latin America and the Caribbean. In: Challenges No. 2. ECLAC-UNICEF; 2006. Available from: http://www.unicef.org/lac/Desafiosnutricion%2813%29.pdf

[10] Food and Agriculture Organization. (2015). Regional Overview of Food Insecurity: Latin America and the Caribbean. Retrieved from the Food and Agriculture Organizarion webstie: http://www.fao.org/3/a-i4636e.pdf

[11] Food and Agriculture Organization. Crecimiento económico, hambre y malnutrición. In: El estado de la inseguridad alimentaria en el mundo 2012. Rome: Food and Agriculture Organization; 2012. pp. 15-29

[12] Galicia L, Grajeda R, López de Romaña D. Nutrition situation in Latin America and the Caribbean: current scenario, past trends and data gaps. Rev Panam Salud Pública. 2016;**40**(2):104-113

[13] World Food Programme. Conferencia regional ministerial. Hacia la erradicación de la desnutrición infantil en América Latina y el Caribe. Panamá: World Food Programme; 2008

[14] Galván M, Amigo H. Programas destinados a disminuir la desnutrición crónica. Una revisión en América Latina. En Archivos Latinoamericanos de Nutrición. 2007;57(4). Disponible en: http://www.researchgate.net/profile/Marcos_Galvan/publication/239613480_Programas_destinados_a_disminuir_la_desnutricin_crnica._Una_revisin_en_America_Latina/links/004635294a45e871e7000000.pdf

[15] Headey D, Hoddinott J, Ali D, Tesfaye R, Dereje M. The Other Asian Enigma: Explaining the Rapid Reduction of Undernutrition in Bangladesh. World Development. 2015;**66**:749-7621. DOI: 10.1016/j.worlddev.2014.09.022

[16] UNICEF. Strategy for improved nutrition of children and women in developing countries. New York: UNICEF; 1990 Retrieved from: https://digitallibrary.un.org/record/227230#:~:text=UNICEF%3B-UNICEF.%20Executive%20Board%20(1990%20sess.%20%3A%20New%20York),-1990

[17] UNICEF. Improving Child Nutrition. The Achievable Imperative for Global Progress. New York: UNICEF. 2013. Retrieved from: file:///Users/margaritamanos/Downloads/NutritionReport_April2013_Final_29.pdf

[18] Engle P, Menon P, Haddad L. Care and Nutrition: Concepts and Measurement. Washington, DC: International Food Policy Research Institute; 1999

[19] Wilma F. Diagnóstico de la situación alimentaria nutricional y de salud de la población ecuatoriana menor de cinco años. Quito: Consejo Nacional de Desarrollo; 1988

[20] CEPAR. Encuesta Demográfica y de Salud Materna e Infantil. Quito: Centro de Estudios de Población y Desarrollo Social. 2005

[21] World Bank. Nutritional Insufficiency in Ecuador. Causes, Consequences and Solutions. Washington: World Bank; 2007

[22] Freire WB, Ramírez MJ, Belmont P, Mendieta MJ, Silva KM, Romero MR. Resumen Ejecutivo. Tomo 1. Encuesta Nacional de Salud y Nutrición ENSANUT-ECU 2011-2013 (Report from the Ministry of Public Health and the National Institute of Statistics and Census). 2014

[23] Carlos L, Freire W, Lutter C, editors. Equidad desde el principio: Situación nutricional de los niños ecuatorianos. Washington, DC: OPS-MSP; 2001

[24] Larrea C, Freire W. Social inequality and child malnutrition in four Andean countries. Rev Panam Salud Publica. 2002;**11**(5/6):356-364. Retrieved from: http://www.scielosp.org/scielo.php?script=sci_arttext&pid=S1020-49892002000500010&lng=pt&nrm=iso&tlng=enPublicHealth,11(5/6),356-364

[25] MIES. Situación de la desnutrición crónica en niños y niñas de los Dervicios de Desarrollo Infantil Integral del Ecuador. Ministerio de Inclusión Económica y Social: Quito; 2015 Retrieved from: http://sitp.pichincha.gob.ec/repositorio/diseno_paginas/archivos/Desnutricion%20investigacion%20MIES.pdf

[26] Creswell J. A Concise Introduction to Mixed Methods Research. California: SAGE Publications; 2015

[27] Hernández R, Collado C, Lucio P. Metodología de la investigación. México D.F., SA: Mc Graw W-Hill / Interamericana Editores; 2014

[28] INEC. National Institute of Statistics and Census. Bases de datos: Condiciones de Vida (ECV) 2006 [Data file and code book]. 2006. Retrieved from: http://www.ecuadorencifras.gob.ec/condiciones-de-vida-ecv-bases-de-datos/

[29] INEC. National Institute of Statistics and Census. Encuesta de condiciones de

vida 2013-2014. Base primaria [Data file and code book]. 2014. Retrieved from: http://www.ecuadorencifras.gob.ec// documentos/web-inec/ECV/ECV_2015/

[30] INEC. National Institute of Statistics and Census. Bases de datos: Condiciones de Vida (ECV) 1998 [Data file and code book]. 1998. Retrieved from http://www.ecuadorencifras.gob.ec/ condiciones-de-vida-ecv-bases-de-datos/

[31] INEC. National Institute of Statistics and Census. Bases de datos: Condiciones de Vida (ECV) 1999 [Data file and code book]. 1999. Retrieved from http://www.ecuadorencifras.gob.ec/ condiciones-de-vida-ecv-bases-de-datos/

[32] INEC. National Institute of Statistics and Census. Bases de Datos: Encuesta Nacional de Ingresos y Gastos de los Hogares Urbanos y Rurales 2004 [Data file and code book]. 2004. Retrieved from: http://www.ecuadorencifras.gob. ec//encuesta-nacional-de-ingresos-y-gastos-de-los-hogares-urbanos-y-rurales-bases-de-datos/

[33] Carrasco F. Actualización de datos sobre desnutrición crónica Infantil en el Ecuador, 2006-2014. Inédito: Documento de trabajo; 2015

[34] Central Bank of Ecuador. Economic Figures of Ecuador. Quito: BCE; December 2014. Available from: https://contenido. bce.fin.ec/documentos/Estadisticas/ SectorReal/Previsiones/IndCoyuntura/ CifrasEconomicas/cie201412.pdf

[35] Ministry of Finance. Justificative Proforma General Budget of the State 2015. Quito: Undersecretariat of Budget; 2015

[36] Naranjo M. Sistemas de protección social en América latina y el Caribe. Ecuador. Santiago de Chile: United Nations; 2013

[37] Ponce J. Inequality of Income in Ecuador: An Analysis of the 1990s and 2000s. Quito: FLACSO; 2011

[38] Banco Mundial. Indicadores: PIB per capita Ecuador 1986-2014. 2014. Available from: http://datos. bancomundial.org/indicador/NY.GDP. PCAP.CD [Visita el 15.05.2014. 14:15]

[39] INEC. National Institute of Statistics and Census. Reporte de pobreza por consumo 2006-2014. Quito: National Institute of Statistics and Census; 2016

[40] Ordóñez A, Samman E, Mariotti C, Borja I. Compartiendo los frutos del progreso Reducción de la pobreza en Ecuador. Londres: Overseas Development Institute; 2015

[41] Banco Central del Ecuador (BCE). Cifras económicas del Ecuador. Quito: BCE; Diciembre 2014. Available from: https://contenido.bce.fin.ec/documentos/ Estadisticas/SectorReal/Previsiones/ IndCoyuntura/CifrasEconomicas/ cie201412.pdf

[42] Martínez L. La Agricultura Familiar en el Ecuador. Informe del Proyecto Análisis de la Pobreza y Desigualdad en América Latina Rural (Desarrollo con Cohesión Territorial Working Paper No. 147). 2013. Retrieved from: http:// portalsiget.net/ArchivosSIGET/recursos/ Archivos/1682015_AgriculturaFamiliarE. pdf

[43] Pérez Sáinz JP. "Postneoliberalism" and Social Inequalities in the Andes: Reflections and Hypotheses on the Venezuelan, Bolivian, and Ecuadorian Cases in A Moment of Equality for Latin America? In: Fritz B, Lavinas L, editors. Challenges for Redistribution. 2016. pp. 53-76

[44] INEC. National Institute of Statistics and Census. Reporte de pobreza por

consumo en Ecuador. 2006-2014. Quito: INEC. 2016. Retrieved from: https://www.ecuadorencifras.gob.ec/documentos/web-inec/Bibliotecas/Libros/reportePobreza.pdf

[45] Babu S, Sanyal P. Food Security, Poverty and Nutrition Policy Analysis. 1st ed. Cambridge: Academic Press; 2009

[46] INEC. National Survey of Income and Expenses of Ecuadorian Households - ENIGHU 2003-2004. Quito: National Institute of Statistics and Census. Retrieved from: https://www.ecuadorencifras.gob.ec/encuesta-nacional-de-ingresos-y-gastos-de-los-hogares-urbanos-enighu-2004/

[47] INEC. National Survey of Income and Expenses of Ecuadorian Households - ENIGHU 2011-2012. Quit[1]o: National Institute of Statistics and Census. Retrieved from: https://anda.inec.gob.ec/anda/index.php/catalog/291

[48] INEC. Database Censo de población y Vivienda 2010. Quito: National Institute of Statistics and Census. Retrieved from: https://www.ecuadorencifras.gob.ec/base-de-datos-censo-de-poblacion-y-vivienda/

[49] INEC National Survey of Employment-ENEMDU 2007 – 2014. Quito: National Institute of Statistics and Census

Section 3

Breastfeeding and COVID Pandemic

Chapter 4

Breastfeeding during COVID Pandemic

Ka-Huen Yip, Mei-Kuen Chow, Yuk-Chiu Yip and Wai-King Tsui

Abstract

As new mothers are understandably concerned about COVID-19 and its high rate of infection, they are often unsure if they should breastfeed their infants. In general, hospitals do not allow direct breastfeeding by mothers with an active infection of SARS-CoV-2. Some neonatal units in Hong Kong maintain safe practices by isolating infants and mothers for at least 7 to 14 days, even if the infant remains SARS-CoV-2 negative. During isolation, mothers encourage the expression of milk to maintain milk duct patency and to prepare for lactation when they and their infants are discharged. Infants are fed formula milk by cup feeding with added supplements based on the recommended daily feeding volume for neonates and their appetite during hospitalization. At present, data that indicates COVID-19 could be transmitted from mother to infant postnatally through breastfeeding are insufficient. Major organizations recommend that mothers should breastfeed exclusively for the first 6 months, and thereafter continue to provide their infants with breast milk up until the age of two or beyond. With new findings arising from research, updated information is important to reassure mothers that breastfeeding at home during the COVID-19 pandemic is safe and recommended for both the mother and the infant.

Keywords: breastfeeding, COVID-19, mothers, mother to child, SARS-cov-2

1. Introduction

The Coronavirus disease (COVID-19) pandemic persisted for over 24 months, following its initial onset in late 2019. It transformed the everyday lives of people worldwide, specifically as they now had to adopt defensive behaviors and habits to prevent the spread of the infection [1, 2]. According to the World Health Organization (WHO), by April 2022, over 492 million cases of COVID-19 were confirmed globally with over 6 million deaths [3]. Worldwide, various preventive and control measures were implemented. In Hong Kong, measures included compulsory quarantine of people entering the city, mandatory use of face masks in public places and on public transport, social distancing in restaurants, cinemas, and all other areas accessible to the public [4, 5].

However, a potentially negative impact on the emergent parent-infant relationship has resulted from these preventative and restrictive measures. Mobile phones of many new parents in the rapidly changing and health-threatening COVID-19 pandemic were flooded with mixed information from various online media and health organizations [5]. This information did not always align but often even contradicted each other. It is well known that breastfeeding is best for newborn infants [6]. As new mothers are concerned about the spread of COVID-19, they remain at home and refrain from taking their infants outside. They have many queries around the care practices they should follow when it comes to their infants during the pandemic. These parents are often equally worried about if they should still breastfeed their infants. Regular updates on the correct caring guidelines and support from the community is required to reassure new mothers regarding the safety of breastfeeding [7].

COVID-19 is a life-threatening and contagious disease. At present, data that indicates that COVID-19 could be vertically transmitted from mother to infant in utero or postnatally through direct respiratory inhalation or breastfeeding are insufficient [8]. These concerns led to anecdotal reports in international news and social media posts of mothers giving birth without a partner or support of a doula that sometimes suggested that breastfeeding is unsafe [9, 10]. In contrast, breastfeeding was promoted in Hong Kong [11, 12]. Appropriate promotions like these and the spread of updated information are particularly helpful to new mothers and their families. It not only enhances their understanding of the various care components but also reassures mothers that breastfeeding at home during the COVID-19 pandemic is safe and beneficial for both the mother and the infant. Breast milk is considered to be the ultimate mixture when it comes to ensuring the strength of a newborn's immunity.

2. Infant feeding policy and practice

Breast milk is ideal food for newborns. It is safe, convenient and provides the most important nutrients and energy for newborns. It also contains antibodies that come from the mother which help prevent illnesses in infants and assists in protecting them from contracting childhood illnesses. Breastmilk promotes the development of sensory and cognitive skills, as well as a strong immune system that protects against chronic or infectious diseases in the infant [13–15]. Exclusively breastfeeding reduces the risk of infant mortality due to common childhood illnesses such as diarrhea or pneumonia, and helps them recover faster [16].

Breastfeeding reduces waste and the need for other resources like bottles and formula. In addition to being more environmentally friendly, this also aids families who struggle financially. They can now distribute these savings to other areas of family life. Specially for the mother reduces the risk of breast and ovarian cancer. The WHO recommends starting to breastfeed as early as 1 h after birth [17].

2.1 Feeding policy

In Hong Kong, most of the hospitals would recommend that all normal or low-risk infants be exposed to skin-to-skin contact on the mother's chest immediately after birth and that feeding should start within 5 min [18]. All mothers are encouraged to hold their infants in a calm environment and try to feed them without rushing the process [19]. If mother and infant cannot initiate feeding after birth, it is re-initiated as soon as the mother and infant's conditions are stabilized or more conducive to it [20]. Early initiation of breastfeeding when both the mother and infant are ready is essential [21]. This critical period has now become a luxury only afforded to the breastfeeding mother who tested negative for the severe acute respiratory syndrome coronavirus 2 (SARS-CoV-2), as the health care providers combat the fifth wave of COVID-19. These mothers are lucky to bond with their infant without separation during their postpartum period while they are hospitalized.

If the mother and infant are separated because of special care, the mother should be instructed on how to initiate and how to maintain breastfeeding by manual expression. Generally, this is initiated within 6 h after delivery, then breast milk is expressed every 3–4 h, or obtained using a breast pump at regular intervals (approximately every 3 h after lactating starts). Mothers should be advised to feed their infants with expressed breast milk (if feeding is allowed) and encouraged to breastfeed as soon as the infant's physical condition allows it. During the COVID-19 pandemic, certain arrangements were created to prevent cross-infections. Since breastfeeding constitutes a close contact situation, the likelihood of transmitting the virus may increase substantially when aerosol-generating procedures are performed [22, 23]. Despite this, studies have suggested very low rates of vertical/peripartum transmission [22–24]. In general, hospitals do not allow direct breastfeeding by mothers who test positive or who are considered as active carriers. Discussions with parents about the risks versus the benefits of expressed breast milk are desperately needed. Visitation by parents is generally not allowed if mothers have active or are suspected of being infected with COVID-19 [25–27].

The results of studies indicated that the neonatal units of some public hospitals in Hong Kong, had zero cross-infection between patients and newborns [28–31]. According to these studies, most units in public hospitals perform nasopharyngeal aspirates/throat swabs (NPA/TS) to test for SARS-CoV2 and reverse transcription polymerase chain reaction (RT-PCR) tests at birth, on day 1 and day 2–3 and then again some time approximately before the estimated discharge date or before step-down from designated airborne infection isolation rooms (AIIR) [29]. Most units consult microbiology experts and laboratory results to help with the interpretation of the aforementioned tests [28]. However, some units investigate neonatal antibodies for SARS-CoV-2 on day 0–1 by testing the infants blood and also routinely test PCR anywhere from 1 week and again around the time the infant is a month old to check for any possible cases of late positivity [30, 31].

Some units maintain safe practices by isolating infants and mothers for at least 7 to 14 days, even if the infant remains SARS-CoV-2 negative [32]. There is no consensus regarding the minimum isolation period for infants of recovered mothers and the use of anti-SARS-CoV-2 antibody testing in the management of these infants. During isolation, mothers encourage the expression of milk to maintain mild duct patency and prepare for lactation when they are discharged with their infants [33]. Infants are fed formular milk with cup feeding and supplements based on the recommended daily feeding volume for neonates and their appetite during hospitalization.

Hong Kong is facing a backlash from healthcare professionals and parents after starting ambush-mode lockdowns and separating parents from infant and toddler in a hopeless effort to contain a fifth wave of COVID-19 pandemic in the densely populated city. The general units of public hospitals do not allow direct breastfeeding by active mothers against WHO advice. Discussion with parents regarding risks versus benefits of expressed breast milk (EBM) is required. Active or suspected mothers are recommended not direct breastfeeding. EBM may be considered after careful discussion of risks versus benefits with parents and appropriate precautions made regarding expression, transport, and storage. Recovered mothers not recommended with direct breastfeeding if separation is required but EBM encouraged.

However, it requires to discuss with local infection control teams to ascertain optimal methods of handling EBM such as double bags, and separation of freezer storage.

Health providers should encourage breastfeeding whenever possible, emphasizing the benefits of adequate infant nutrition for all newborns. Skin-to-skin contact, or Kangaroo mother care should be allowed when mothers have no contraindication to care for their infants.

3. The background of the infant feeding

Infant feeding is important for infant survival and healthy growth. The primary infant feeding methods for infants under 6 months of age are breastfeeding and bottle feeding. Breastfeeding is the ideal feeding mode for both mothers and infants.

Breastfeeding provides health benefits to bother mothers and infants [34, 35]. Major organizations recommend that mothers should breastfeed exclusively for the first 6 months, and thereafter continue to provide their infants with breast milk for up to 2 years of age or beyond [17, 36–38]. According to the WHO, optimal breastfeeding is critical and could save the lives of over 820,000 infants and children under the age of 5 years annually [39].

Breastfeeding has important short- and long-term benefits for both infants and mothers [40, 41]. In addition to health benefits, breastfeeding is the most ecologically sustainable way to feed infants and provides substantial cost savings to families [42]. Global public health recommendations stated that infants should be exclusively breastfed for the first 6 months of life to achieve optimal growth, development, and health [43]. Thereafter, it is a norm to meet the evolving nutritional requirements of this vulnerable group for their well-being and provider nutritionally adequate and safe complementary foods while breastfeeding for up to 2 years of age or beyond [44]. Exclusive breastfeeding from birth is possible, except for a limited special healthcare needs situation [45].

Despite this recommendation, breastfeeding rates vary widely; in the United Kingdom, the exclusively breastfed at 1 week of age is 46%, and at <1% at 6 months [46].

In Australia, the National Infant Feeding Survey, a large-scale data result indicated that breastfeeding was initiated for 96% of children aged 0–2 years and approximately 69% of infants were still receiving breast milk at 4 months of age in 2010. However, only 39% were exclusively breastfed for 3 months, and only 15% were exclusively breastfed to five completed months of age [47].

In Hong Kong, although the Department of Health introduced supportive breastfeeding initiatives that led to an increase in breastfeeding mothers in 2019 (up to 87.2% of mothers) [48], many mothers give up the practice within just a few months [49].

The main reason these women were eager to discontinue breastfeeding in the first 3 months after birth were work responsibilities [50]. Maternity leave in the city usually lasts for 10 weeks [51] and flexible working arrangements are difficult to negotiate with many employers.

Since 2015, the Hong Kong government has been trying to fight discrimination. Food and Health Bureau (FHB) encouraged government and private facilities to implement "breastfeeding-friendly workplace" policies and measures to facilitate new mothers to continue breastfeeding after return to work [52]. Moreover, Professor

Sophia Chan Siu-chee (Secretary for FHB, HKSAR) issued regulations for employers who wish to create a breastfeeding-friendly workplace in Hong Kong [53].

4. Pregnancy and breastfeeding during the COVID-19 pandemic

COVID-19 is an infectious disease that was declared a public health emergency of international concern by the WHO [54]. Their main concern is whether breastfeeding by mothers infected with COVID-19 is safe, and whether the virus or antibodies can be transmitted from mother to baby through milk [55].

Pregnant and/or breastfeeding women have not been included in studies to determine how well COVID-19 vaccines work or how safe they are [56]. Especially in Hong Kong, up till now, there are no study conducted based on the pregnancy women and breastfeeding issues.

Only based on other similar infectious diseases, we believe the risks that come with vaccination will probably be low [56]. Therefore, while we wait for more information, each mother and the health professional should discuss what choice fits their situation best. As for breastfeeding, little or none of these vaccine components would ever reach the milk compartment, or even be transferred into human milk. Even if they were the infant would simply digest them like any other protein, that the present group of vaccines is probably going to be quite safe for breastfeeding mothers [57]. The infant may even gain a small amount of maternal IgG in the breastmilk, which may even be beneficial [57, 58].

In before, breastfeeding by mothers infected with SARS-CoV-2 is highly recommended for infants if the health of the mother and infant allow for it. Direct breastfeeding and preservation of appropriate protective measures should be encouraged [59]. If the mother's health condition does not allow direct breastfeeding, infants should be fed pumped breast milk or donor milk.

Emerging data indicate that people with comorbidities and those aged over 60 years have an increased risk of severe respiratory disease and death [60]. Pregnant women do not appear to be adversely affected. Pregnant women with severe respiratory infections, such as pneumonia, are usually associated with adverse health outcomes for both women and babies, consisting of eclampsia, increased intensity of maternal mortality, and preterm birth [61].

Findings from Italy demonstrated women's expectations and concerns regarding childbirth before and after the onset of the pandemic. Women were more concerned about the health of others than their own; they had a history of psychological distress that was significantly more overwhelmed by the pandemic; expressions of emotions and psychological constructs around childbirth dramatically changed before and after the onset of COVID-19 [62].

Before the pandemic, most women associated the fear of childbirth with constructs related to physical pain, the commitment of childbirth, the emotion of finally being able to meet the child (joy, happiness, serenity), and a sense of impatience was more closely related to stress and anxiety in this situation [62, 63]. This phenomenon is well known by women and healthcare professionals, such as midwives, worldwide and is considered part of the early physiological anxiety that allows women to prepare for the moment of childbirth in the best possible way [64]. During the pandemic, the change in response was startling: fear no longer correlated with anticipation, impatience, joy, and encounter, but with sadness, loneliness, inability, a sense of isolation, and confinement [62].

The COVID-19 pandemic resulted in lockdowns in some countries such as the United Kingdom and the United States, and the resulting social distancing measures led to a decrease in breastfeeding support systems available to women [19, 65]. Some hospitals separate mothers and babies in hospitals, while decreasing face-to-face professional support. Peer support for mothers and their babies was also removed. Meanwhile, new families were confined to their homes, separated from families, and any other support networks. Therefore, breastfeeding is best supported by practices that keep the mother and baby together, high-quality professional and peer-to-peer support, positive maternal well-being, and understanding the impact of the pandemic on the ability to breastfeed [19, 66]. Despite, 27% of mothers hoping to have support, they instead faced many barriers stemming from lockdown and associated measures, resulting in some discontinuing breastfeeding before they were actually ready. The influence of the lockdown and other factors impacted their decision to continue or to stop breastfeeding, including low socioeconomic status, living atmospheres, and ethnic differences. Healthcare professionals need to be vigorous in their endeavors to understand and provide support to these vulnerable women, who may be grieving the loss of their ability to breastfeed and who are affected by their negative experiences. It is important to learn from women with positive experiences of caring for their infants during the pandemic to demonstrate what would be considered better support if a similar crisis occurs.

5. Conclusion

Breast milk is an ideal food source for newborns. Breastmilk promotes sensory and cognitive development and protects defenseless infants against any chronic or infectious diseases due to the antibodies present in it. Exclusively breastfeeding reduces infant mortality related to common childhood illnesses, such as diarrhea or pneumonia, and helps hasten their recovery during an illness. The COVID-19 pandemic raised issues regarding the safety of breastfeeding. Mothers with active, suspected, or past COVID-19 results must follow certain precautions and guidelines to prevent cross-infections, since breastfeeding constitutes a close contact situation. In general, hospitals do not allow mothers with an active infection with SARS-CoV-2 to directly breastfeed their babies. Some neonatal units in Hong Kong enforce safe practices by isolating infants and mothers for at least 7 to 14 days, even if the infant remains SARS-CoV-2 negative. If the mother and infant are separated due to their need for special care, the mother should be encouraged to express milk to maintain milk duct patency and to prepare her for lactation when they are discharged with their infants. During isolation, infants are cup fed formula milk with additional supplements based on the recommended daily feeding volume and requirements for neonates and their appetite during hospitalization. Regular updates on the correct caring guidelines and support from the community is required to reassure new mothers regarding the feasibility of direct breastfeeding during and following the pandemic. Major organizations recommend that mothers should breastfeed exclusively for the first 6 months, and thereafter continue to provide their infants with breast milk until they are 2 years old or beyond.

Acknowledgements

This research was funded by the Institute Development Grant (IDG) [Reference no.: IDG210201] of Caritas Institute of Higher Education.

Conflict of interest

The authors declare that there are no conflicts of interest.

Notes/thanks/other declarations

None.

Author details

Ka-Huen Yip*, Mei-Kuen Chow, Yuk-Chiu Yip and Wai-King Tsui
School of Health Sciences, Caritas Institute of Higher Education, Hong Kong, China

*Address all correspondence to: khyip@cihe.edu.hk

References

[1] Kickbusch I, Leung GM, Bhutta ZA, Matsoso MP, Ihekweazu C, Abbasi K. Covid-19: How a virus is turning the world upside down. BMJ. 2020;**369**: m1336. DOI: 10.1136/bmj.m1336

[2] Lades LK, Laffan K, Daly M, Delaney L. Daily emotional well-being during the COVID-19 pandemic. British Journal of Health Psychology. 2020;**25**(4):902-911. DOI: 10.1111/bjhp.12450

[3] World Health Organization. WHO Coronavirus (COVID-19) Dashboard [Internet]. 2022. Available from: https://covid19.who.int/ [Accessed: April 7, 2022]

[4] Family Health Services, Department of Health. Health advice on Coronavirus Disease (COVID-19). The Government of the Hong Kong Special Administrative Region [Internet]. 2021. Available from: https://www.fhs.gov.hk/english/news/nCov2019/ [Accessed: March 11, 2022]

[5] Food and Health Bureau. The Government of the Hong Kong Special Administrative Region. Prevention and control of novel coronavirus infection in Hong Kong [Internet]. 2020. Available from: https://www.legco.gov.hk/yr19-20/english/counmtg/papers/cm20200219p-e.pdf [Accessed: March 11, 2022]

[6] McFadden A, Gavine A, Renfrew MJ, Wade A, Buchanan P, Taylor JL, et al. Support for healthy breastfeeding mothers with healthy term babies. Cochrane Database Sys Rev. 2017;**2**(2):CD001141. DOI: 10.1002/14651858.CD001141.pub5

[7] Gavine A, Mcfadden A, Macgillivray S, Renfrew MJ. Evidence reviews for the ten steps to successful breastfeeding initiative. JHV. 2017;**5**(8):378-380. DOI: 10.12968/johv.2017.5.8.378

[8] Juan J, Gil MM, Rong Z, Zhang Y, Yang H, Poon LC. Effects of coronavirus disease 2019 (COVID-19) on maternal, perinatal and neonatal outcomes: Systematic review. Ultrasound in Obstetrics & Gynecology. 2020;**56**:15-27. DOI: 10.1002/uog.22088

[9] The Guardian. 'There are more births in the car park': A midwife's experience of the Covid-19 crisis [Internet]. 2020. Available from: https://www.theguardian.com/society/2020/jun/04/more-births-car-park-midwifes-experience-covid-19-crisis [Accessed: March 11, 2022]

[10] Pramono A, Dahlen H, Desborough J, Smith JP. Separating mothers with COVID-19 from their newborns does more harm than good. The Conversation. 2020. Available from: https://theconversation.com/separating-mothers-with-covid-19-from-their-newborns-does-more-harm-than-good-141291 [Accessed: March 11, 2022]

[11] The Government of the Hong Kong Special Administrative Region. World Breastfeeding Week promotes collaboration in support of breastfeeding [Internet]. 2021. Available from: https://www.info.gov.hk/gia/general/202108/03/P2021080200536.htm [Accessed: March 11, 2022]

[12] UNICEF UK. UNICEF UK Baby Friendly Initiative Statement on Infant Feeding during the Coronavirus (COVID-19) Outbreak [Internet]. 2021. Available from: https://www.unicef.org.uk/babyfriendly/wp-content/uploads/

sites/2/2020/04/Unicef-UK-Baby-Friendly-Initiative-statement-on-infant-feeding-during-the-Covid-19-outbreak.pdf [Accessed: March 11, 2022]

[13] Davidson EL, Ollerton RL. Partner behaviours improving breastfeeding outcomes: An integrative review. Women and Birth. 2020;**33**(1):e15-e23. DOI: 10.1016/j.wombi.2019.05.010

[14] Duijts L, Jaddoe VWV, Hofman A, Moll HA. Prolonged and exclusive breastfeeding reduces the risk of infectious diseases in infancy. Pediatrics. 2010;**126**(1):e18-e25. DOI: 10.1542/peds.2008-3256

[15] Mututho LN, Kiboi WK, Mucheru PK. Factors associated with exclusive breastfeeding in Kenya: A systematic review. International Journal of Community Medicine and Public Health. 2017;**4**(12):4358-4362. DOI: 10.18203/2394-6040.ijcmph 20175305

[16] World Health Organization. Newsroom, Fact sheets, Detail [Internet]. 2018. Available from: https://www.who.int/news-room/fact-sheets/detail/diarrhoea [Accessed: March 11, 2022]

[17] World Health Organization. Breastfeeding [Internet]. 2022. Available from: https://www.who.int/health-topics/breastfeeding [Accessed: March 11, 2022]

[18] Tarrant M, Fong DYT, Wu KM, Lee ILY, Wong EMY, Sham A, et al. Breastfeeding and weaning practices among Hong Kong mothers: A prospective study. BMC Pregnancy and Childbirth. 2010;**10**:27. DOI: 10.1186/1471-2393-10-27

[19] Brown A, Shenker N. Experiences of breastfeeding during COVID-19: Lessons for future practical and emotional support. Maternal & Child Nutrition. 2021;**17**(1):e13088. DOI: 10.1111/mcn.13088

[20] Tran HT, Nguyen TT, Mathisen R. The use of human donor milk. BMJ. 2020;**371**:m4243. DOI: 10.1136/bmj.m4243

[21] Davie P, Chilcot J, Chang YS, Norton S, Hughes LD, Bick D. Effectiveness of social-psychological interventions at promoting breastfeeding initiation, duration and exclusivity: A systematic review and meta-analysis. Health Psychology Review. 2020;**14**(4):449-485. DOI: 10.1080/17437199.2019.1630293

[22] Chen H, Guo J, Wang C, Luo F, Yu X, Zhang W, et al. Clinical characteristics and intrauterine vertical transmission potential of COVID-19 infection in nine pregnant women: A retrospective review of medical records. The Lancet. 2020;**395**(10226):809-815. DOI: 10.1016/S0140-6736(20)30360-3

[23] Gale C, Quigley MA, Placzek A, Knight M, Ladhani S, Draper ES, et al. Characteristics and outcomes of neonatal SARS-CoV-2 infection in the UK: A prospective national cohort study using active surveillance. Lancet Child Adolesc Health. 2020;**5**(2):113-121. DOI: 10.1016/S2352-4642(20)30342-4

[24] Zeng L, Xia S, Yuan W, Yan K, Xiao F, Shao J, et al. Neonatal early-onset infection with SARS-CoV-2 in 33 neonates born to mothers with COVID-19 in Wuhan, China. JAMA Pediatrics. 2020;**174**(7):722-725. DOI: 10.1001/jamapediatrics.2020.0878

[25] Amatya S, Corr TE, Gandhi CK, Glass KM, Kresch MJ, Mujsce DJ, et al. Management of newborns exposed to mothers with confirmed or suspected COVID-19. American Journal of Perinatology. 2020;**40**(7):987-996. DOI: 10.1038/s41372-020-0695-0

[26] Chandrasekharan P, Vento M, Trevisanuto D, Partridge E, Underwood MA, Wiedeman J, et al. NeonatalresuscitationandPostresuscitation Care of Infants Born to mothers with suspected or confirmed SARS-CoV-2 infection. American Journal of Perinatology. 2020;**37**(8):813-824. DOI: 10.1055/s-0040-1709688

[27] Kotlar B, Gerson E, Petrillo S, Langer A, Tiemeier H. The impact of the COVID-19 pandemic on maternal and perinatal health: A scoping review. Reproductive Health. 2021;**18**(10):1-39. DOI: 10.1186/s12978-021-01070-6

[28] Leung TF, Ng PC, Cheng FWT, Lyon DJ, So KW, Hon EKL, et al. Infection control for SARS in a tertiary paediatric Centre in Hong Kong. The Journal of Hospital Infection. 2004;**56**(3):215-222. DOI: 10.1016/j.jhin.2003.11.004

[29] Ng PC, So KW, Leung TF, Cheng FWT, Lyon DJ, Wong W, et al. Infection control for SARS in a tertiary neonatal Centre. Archives of Disease in Childhood. Fetal and Neonatal Edition. 2003;**88**(5):F405-F409. DOI: 10.1136/fn.88.5.F405

[30] Ng PC. Infection control measures for COVID-19 in the labour suite and neonatal unit. Neonatology. 2020;**117**(2):141-143. DOI: 10.1159/000508002

[31] Shek CC, Ng PC, Fung GPG, Cheng FWT, Chan PKS, Peiris MJS, et al. Infants born to mothers with severe acute respiratory syndrome. Pediatrics. 2003;**112**(4):e254-e254. DOI: 10.1542/peds.112.4.e254

[32] Salvatore CM, Han JY, Acker KP, Tiwari P, Jin J, Brandler M, et al. Neonatal management and outcomes during the COVID-19 pandemic: An observation cohort study. The Lancet Child & Adolescent Health. 2020;**4**(10):721-727. DOI: 10.1016/S2352-4642(20)30235-2

[33] Centers for Disease Control and Prevention [CDC] Breastfeeding: Supporting evidence for maternity practices in infant nutrition and care (mPINC) [Internet]. Available from: https://www.cdc.gov/breastfeeding/pdf/mpinc/supporting-evidence-for-mPINC-508.pdf [Accessed: April 7, 2022]

[34] Brown A. Breastfeeding as a public health responsibility: A review of the evidence. Journal of Human Nutrition and Dietetics. 2017;**30**(6):759-770. DOI: 10.1111/jhn.12496

[35] Ng CA, Ho JJ, Lee ZH. The effect of rooming-in on duration of breastfeeding: A systematic review of randomised and non-randomised prospective controlled studies. PLoS One. 2019;**14**(4):e0215869. DOI: 10.1371/journal.pone.0215869

[36] Centers for Disease Control and Prevention [CDC] Breastfeeding report card [Internet]. 2021 Available from: https://www.cdc.gov/breastfeeding/data/reportcard.htm [Accessed: February 28, 2022]

[37] US Department of Agriculture; US Department of Health and Human Services. Dietary guidelines for Americans, 2020-2025. 9th ed. 2020 [Internet]. Available from: https://www.dietaryguidelines.gov/ [Accessed: March 11, 2022]

[38] World Health Organization. Breastfeeding and COVID-19 [Internet]. 2020. Available from: https://www.who.int/publications/i/item/WHO-2019-nCoV-Sci_Brief-Breastfeeding-2020.1 [Accessed: March 11, 2022]

[39] World Health Organization. Infant and young child feeding fact sheet

[Internet]. 2022. Available from: https://apps.who.int/nutrition/publications/infantfeeding/en/index.html [Accessed: March 11, 2022]

[40] Perrine CG, Scanlon KS, Li R, Odom E, Grummer-Strawn LM. Baby-friendly hospital practices and meeting exclusive breastfeeding intention. Pediatrics. 2012;**130**(1):54-60. DOI: 10.1542/peds.2011-3633

[41] The Government of the Hong Kong Special Administrative Region. Press releases: World Breastfeeding Week 2019 calls for community support for breastfeeding (with photos) [Internet]. 2019. Available from: https://www.info.gov.hk/gia/general/201907/27/P2019072600650.htm [Accessed: March 11, 2022]

[42] Schmied V, Burns E, Sheehan A. Place of sanctuary: An appreciative inquiry approach to discovering how communities support breastfeeding and parenting. International Breastfeeding Journal. 2019;**14**(1):1-14. DOI: 10.1186/s13006-019-0219-8

[43] Smith J, Cattaneo A, Iellamo A, Javanparast S, Atchan M, Gribble K, Hartmann B, Salmon L, Tawia S, Hull N, Linkson M, Blake M, Elliott-Rudder M. Review of effective strategies to promote breastfeeding. The Sax Institute. 2018. Available from: https://apo.org.au/sites/default/files/resource-files/2018-05/apo-nid182256.pdf [Accessed: March 11, 2022]

[44] Greer FR, Sicherer SH, Burks AW. The effects of early nutritional interventions on the development of atopic disease in infants and children: The role of maternal dietary restriction, breastfeeding, hydrolyzed formulas, and timing of introduction of allergenic complementary foods. Pediatrics. 2019;**143**(4):1-11. DOI: 10.1542/peds.2019-0281

[45] Thepha T, Marais D, Bell J, Muangpin S. Perceptions of northeast Thai breastfeeding mothers regarding facilitators and barriers to six-month exclusive breastfeeding: Focus group discussions. International Breastfeeding Journal. 2018;**13**(1):1-10. DOI: 10.1186/s13006-018-0148-y

[46] Fielder C. Determining the influencing factors of a caesarean section birth on breastfeeding. Evid Based Midwifery. 2016;**14**(2):57-63

[47] Australian Institute of Health and Welfare. 2010 Australian National Infant Feeding Survey: Indicator results. Australian Government [Internet]. 2010. Available from: https://www.aihw.gov.au/getmedia/af2fe025-637e-4c09-ba03-33e69f49aba7/13632.pdf.aspx?inline=true [Accessed: March 11, 2022]

[48] Baby Friendly Hospital Initiative Hong Kong Association. World Breastfeeding Week (WBW) [Internet]. 2020. Available from: https://www.babyfriendly.org.hk/wp-content/uploads/2020/08/2020-WBW-Annual-Survey_E_Final.pdf [Accessed: March 11, 2022]

[49] Bai DL, Fong DYT, Tarrant M. Factors associated with breastfeeding duration and exclusivity in mothers returning to paid employment postpartum. Maternal and Child Health Journal. 2015;**19**(5):990-999. DOI: 10.1007/s10995-014-1596-7

[50] Sun K, Chen M, Yin Y, Wu L, Gao L. Why Chinese mothers stop breastfeeding: Mothers' self-reported reasons for stopping during the first six months. Journal of Child Health Care. 2017;**21**(3):353-363. DOI: 10.1177/1367493517719160

[51] Constable N. Tales of two cities: Legislating pregnancy and marriage

among foreign domestic workers in Singapore and Hong Kong. Journal of Ethnic and Migration Studies. 2020;**46**(16):3491-3507. DOI: 10.1080/1369183X.2019.1592403

[52] Equal Opportunities Commission. Let's Build a Breastfeeding-friendly Workplace [Internet]. 2021. Available from: from https://www.eoc.org.hk/eoc/Upload/UserFiles/File/FactSheet/8_Leaflet_on_Breastfeeding_Discrimination_in_the_Workplace_e.pdf [Accessed: March 11, 2022]

[53] Chan SSC. Optimising Breastfeeding Practices: A Public health's Perspective [Internet]. 2014. Available from: https://www3.ha.org.hk/haconvention/hac2014/proceedings/downloads/S2.1.pdf [Accessed: March 11, 2022]

[54] World Health Organization. Statement on the second meeting of the International Health Regulations (2005) Emergency Committee regarding the outbreak of novel coronavirus (2019-nCoV) [Internet]. 2022. Available from: https://www.who.int/news/item/30-01-2020-statement-on-the-second-meeting-of-the-international-health-regulations-(2005)-emergency-committee-regarding-the-outbreak-of-novel-coronavirus-(2019-ncov) [Accessed: March 11, 2022]

[55] Panahi L, Amiri M, Pouy S. Risks of novel coronavirus disease (COVID-19) in pregnancy; a narrative review. Archives of Emergency Medicine. 2020;**8**(1):-e34

[56] Collier AY, McMahan K, Yu J, et al. Immunogenicity of COVID-19 mRNA vaccines in pregnant and lactating women. Journal of the American Medical Association. 2021;**325**(23):2370-2380. DOI: 10.1001/jama.2021.7563

[57] De Rose DU, Salvatori G, Dotta A, Auriti C. SARS-CoV-2 vaccines during pregnancy and breastfeeding: A systematic review of maternal and neonatal outcomes. Viruses. 2022;**14**(3):539. DOI: 10.3390/v14030539

[58] Hale TW. Hale's medications & mothers' milk. In: A Manual of Lactational Pharmacology. 19th ed. New York: Springer Publishing Company; 2021

[59] Pérez-Bermejo M, Peris-Ochando B, Murillo-Llorente MT. COVID-19: Relationship and impact on breastfeeding-a systematic review. Nutrients. 2021;**13**(9):2972. DOI: 10.3390/nu13092972

[60] Onder G, Rezza G, Brusaferro S. Case-fatality rate and characteristics of patients dying in relation to COVID-19 in Italy. Journal of the American Medical Association. 2020;**323**(18):1775-1776. DOI: 10.1001/jama.2020.4683

[61] Chen YH, Keller J, Wang IT, Lin CC, Lin HC. Pneumonia and pregnancy outcomes: A nationwide population-based study. American Journal of Obstetrics and Gynecology. 2012;**207**(4):288-2e1. DOI: 10.1016/j.ajog.2012.08.023

[62] Ravaldi C, Wilson A, Ricca V, Homer C, Vannacci A. Pregnant women voice their concerns and birth expectations during the COVID-19 pandemic in Italy. Women and Birth. 2021;**34**(4):335-343. DOI: 10.1016/j.wombi.2020.07.002

[63] Karavadra B, Stockl A, Prosser-Snelling E, Simpson P, Morris E. Women's perceptions of COVID-19 and their healthcare experiences: A qualitative thematic analysis of national survey of pregnant women in the United Kingdom. BMC Pregnancy and Childbirth. 2020;**20**(1):1-8. DOI: 10.1186/s12884-020-03283-2

[64] Shorey S, Chan V. Lessons from past epidemics and pandemics and a way forward for pregnant women, midwives and nurses during COVID-19 and beyond: A meta-synthesis. Midwifery. 2020;**90**:102821. DOI: 10.1016/j.midw.2020.102821

[65] Latorre G, Martinelli D, Guida P, Masi E, De Benedictis R, Maggio L. Impact of COVID-19 pandemic lockdown on exclusive breastfeeding in non-infected mothers. International Breastfeeding Journal. 2021;**16**(1):1-7. DOI: 10.1186/s130006-021-00382-4

[66] Ingram J, Thomson G, Johnson D, Clarke JL, Trickey H, Hoddinott P, et al. On behalf of the ABA study team. Women's and peer supporters' experiences of an assets-based peer support intervention for increasing breastfeeding initiation and continuation: A qualitative study. Health Expectations. 2020;**23**:622-631. DOI: 10.1111/hex.13042

Section 4

Formula Feeding; Fat Component Safety

Chapter 5

Research of Fat Component Safety and Pre-Clinical Evaluation of Infant Adapted Dry Milk Mixtures Physiological Effect

Ekaterina Yurievna Volf, Inna Vladimirovna Simakova, Andrey Anatolyevich Terentyev, Aleksandr Sergeevich Fedonnikov, Nina Viktorovna Bolotova, Gloria Vladimirovna Guzeeva and Viktor Veniaminovich Zakrevsky

Abstract

The aim of the study deals with determination of fat component safety and quality key indicators of adapted infant dry milk formulas provided by various manufacturers. The most popular in Russia adapted infant dry milk formulas were selected as study objects. It was found that the qualitative composition of the fat component of dry milk mixtures corresponds to the information placed on the package. However none of the samples under study in terms of the average composition of the prevailing fatty acids fully corresponds to human breast milk. The regulation documents of the Customs Union (TR CU 021/2011, TR CU 024/2011, TR CU 033/2013) establish only the organoleptic evaluation of the adapted breast milk formulas quality indicators. Among the fat component safety indicators only the determination of the peroxide value characterizing the accumulation of primary fat oxidation products. It was also found that the peroxide values of the studied mixtures do not exceed the regulated values. Meanwhile the samples of infant milk food made from dry milk mixtures almost all have unsatisfactory organoleptic characteristics. Defects of taste and smell are associated with the accumulation in the original adapted milk mixtures of a significant amount of secondary products of fat oxidation, which in a biological experiment on animals lead to a decrease in the content of leukocytes and a change of its blood count.

Keywords: infant adapted dry milk formulas, safety, fat component, physiological effect, histological pattern

1. Introduction

The optimum food product for an infant in the first months of life is the breastmilk which corresponds to the characteristics of its digestive system and metabolism which ensures the adequate development of an infant's body with a rational diet of a lactating woman. Lactotrophic nutrition (breastfeeding) is the postnatal equivalent of fetal hemotrophic nutrition. It has a unique biological and emotional impact on the health of both mother and baby. All nutrients in human milk are easily absorbed if their composition and ratio correspond to the functional capabilities of the gastrointestinal tract of an infant. After the birth of a child, the "mother-placenta-fetus" system transforms into its postnatal analog "mother-mammary gland-breast milk-infant" with the preservation of the genetic link formed during prenatal development. Thus breastfeeding being an important factor in the formation of health has a multifaceted effect on infants' physical and mental development as well as the formation of their behavior and intellectual development [1, 2].

However, a significant proportion of women by means of various reasons are unable to provide their infant with natural feeding. In these cases, it is important to organize optimum artificial feeding which cannot replace breast milk. But with the proper approach may ensure the correct growth and development of the child [3]. The modern trend of bottle-feeding is connected with the use of specialized industrial baby food products, modern breast milk substitutes, so-called baby "mixtures"—adapted milk formulas. The main goal of its production is the maximal adaptation to the composition and properties of breast milk as well as taking into account the nature of the child's digestion. Approximation of the composition provided by addition of the following components: carbohydrate, mineral, vitamin, protein, and fat [4]. The need for the fat component in an infant is a maximum—44–49% of the energy value of the diet [3]. A number of studies have shown that approximating the composition of mixtures fat components closer to the composition of breast milk can contribute to a more harmonious development of the child and reduce the risk of infection [5, 6], improving the psychoemotional and physical growth and development of children at the age of 4 months [6], improves cognitive development and also has a significant impact on the intellectual development [7, 8]. Therefore, it is extremely important that the child continues to receive the fat component of the optimal composition either with breast milk or with infant formula [9].

One of the expected results of the implementation of global strategies in the field of healthy nutrition is the reduction of alimentary-dependent diseases among children providing them with adequate nutrition from the first days of life. Due to the immaturity of protective mechanisms, physiological and metabolic characteristics of young children, increased hygienic requirements are imposed on the safety and quality of infant food [10].

In the scientific literature, studies of infant formula are widely presented. They are dedicated to their compliance with the requirements of regulatory documents in terms of the quantitative composition of the components of the mixture [11], toxicological safety [12, 13], weight gain of the child, tolerance of the mixture [14]. At the same time, there're a limited number of studies dedicated to the change in the qualitative characteristics of the lipid fraction of infant formula during storage [15, 16]. However, thermal treatment of native raw materials at the stage of spray drying, a sufficiently long shelf life can provoke the oxidation of the fat component which is a potential source of danger to the body. This is due to the fact that during the oxidation process such undesirable oxidation products as glycidol ethers [17–20], epoxides, secondary oxidation products insoluble in petroleum ether are formed which have teratogenic, mutagenic, and carcinogenic effects [21, 22].

Thus, the safety requirements for the fat component of adapted milk formulas, in our opinion, are not sufficiently presented in the legal requirements of the Russian Federation and the Customs Union.

The aim of this work was a pilot study of some indicators of the safety and quality of the fat component of adapted infant dry milk formulas from various manufacturers.

2. Objects of research and research methods

The research was carried out in two stages. At the first stage among the wide range of infant formulas available on the market, the popular in Russia adapted infant dry milk formulas "IS" (Denmark), "IM", "IN", "IL" (Russian Federation), "IX "(Germany) were selected as research objects. The shelf life of infant formula according to the manufacturers' documentary standards is equal to 18 months. The packages purchased through retail chains were unsealed in the initial period of their shelf life—before 6 months of expiration. The study of physical and chemical indicators was carried out immediately after opening the package. Fat for analysis was isolated from dry milk mixtures by the extraction-weight method. In the extracted fat the fatty acid composition was determined by gas-liquid chromatography of fatty acid methyl esters. Methyl esters of fatty acids were prepared according to and the compliance with the average fatty acid composition of the studied mixtures to the composition of human milk was assessed.

The legal requirements of the Customs Union (TR CU 0211/2011, TR CU 033/2013) regulate only organoleptic indicators of the quality indicators of adapted infant dry milk mixtures. However, among the safety indicators of the fat component, it regulates only the determination of the peroxide value, which characterizes the accumulation of primary products of fat oxidation. The peroxide number of the fat component of the mixtures was determined by the iodometric method. Infant milk food for organoleptic analysis was prepared according to the recommendations indicated on the package with a hydromodule of 1–3. Organoleptic analysis was carried out by a descriptive method. All experiments were carried out in triplicate.

At the second stage, *in vivo* experiments were carried out. In vivo biomodels allow obtaining multifactorial data on the effect on various organ systems and the entire body as a whole. The advantages of *in vivo* methods are connected with their adequacy and reliability, a high degree of correlation with the human, and the possibility of a comprehensive evaluation of properties. In this regard, the samples of mixtures were studied with the participation of biomodels which were Wistar rats. The experiment involved six groups of Wistar rats 65 days old with an initial weight of 130–210 g, corresponding to the Minimal Diseases quality standard for the control and experimental groups. In the first experimental group, the usual diet was replaced with mixture 1; in the second experimental group the usual diet was replaced with mixture 2; in the third experimental group the usual diet was replaced with mixture 3; in the fourth experimental group the usual diet was replaced with mixture 4; in the fifth experimental group, the usual diet was replaced with mixture 5 accordingly. Research on animals was carried out in accordance with the "Rules for work on experimental animals", with Directive 2010/63/EU of the European Parliament and of the Council of the European Union of September 22, 2010, on the protection of animals used for scientific purposes, and was carried out on the basis of a certified vivarium of the Scientific and Technological Center of Veterinary hospital and laboratories of the Department of Morphology, Pathology of Animals and Biology of the Saratov State Agrarian University named after N.I. Vavilov. All experimental studies were carried out on groups of clinically healthy rats, formed according to the principle of analogs, taking into account the breed, sex, age, live weight, and clinical condition. The animals were fed for 40 days. During the experiment, the rats were kept in individual cages (10 individuals in each). Before the introduction of the studied mixtures into the diet, animals were kept in quarantine for 21 days (to detect latent forms of diseases) and transferred to the experimental diet in accordance with the experimental plan. After the experiment, the rats were sacrificed by the optimum and universal method which was given anesthesia overdose, also known as the introduction of an anesthetic in a lethal dose (dosage for anesthesia x3), in compliance with the rules of euthanasia for animals (order of the USSR Ministry of Health No. 755 of 08/12/1977), then autopsy was performed. Samples of tissues of the liver, kidneys, spleen, small and large intestines were taken from biomodels, after fixation of which morphological and statistical studies were carried out. From paraffin blocks on a sled microtome model 2712 (Reichert Wien), histological sections with a thickness of 8 μm were obtained, processed according to conventional techniques, and stained with Ehrlich's hematoxylin and eosin, followed by microscopy [23, 24]. The morphological structure was studied on various histological sections. Histological examination of the prepared preparations was carried out under different magnifications with detailed logging and photographing of the studied areas. Microphotography of histological preparations was carried out using a CANON Power Shot A460 IS camera. Statistical processing of the results was carried out using standard methods. The work was carried out on the basis of research laboratories of the Saratov State Agrarian University named after N.I. Vavilov.

Statistical data analysis was carried out using the licensed computer software package STATISTICA 10, StatSoft, Inc. (Series 0411-R) using the methods of biomedical statistics with the calculation of the mean and standard error of the mean. Checking the normality of the distribution of quantitative data was carried out using the Shapiro-Wilks test. For all indicators including behavioral studies, with normally distributed data intergroup comparisons were made using Student's t-test for independent samples at $p < 0.05$.

3. Discussion of the results

Preliminary study of the ready-to-use samples of mixtures showed that almost all samples had an unsatisfactory taste and smell which is characteristic of the relatively oxidized fat components of mixtures. Therefore, for a more complete evaluation of the hydrolysis degree and oxidation of the fat component in the mixtures, the acid number of the released fat was determined by the titrimetric method, the anisidine number was determined by a method based on measuring the optical concentration of the analyzed solution after reaction with an acetic acid solution of paraanisidine. The measurement takes place in the presence of 350 nm waves. The content of secondary oxidation products insoluble in petroleum ether (CIPE) according to an increase in the intensity of the absorption band of ultraviolet radiation at a wavelength of 232 nm, which corresponds to the absorption of conjugated dienechromophores. The content of epoxides was determined according to reactions with concentrated phosphoric acid. All studies were carried out immediately after opening the cans with mixtures.

Determination of the acid number is important for determining the degree of fat hydrolysis. This indicator is of particular importance when analyzing mixtures containing coconut and palm kernel oils, since a soapy aftertaste occurs when the mixture contains appreciable amounts of free lauric acid. In addition, during intensive hydrolysis of fats, di- and monoglycerides accumulate, which, according to modern data, can be precursors of the dangerous toxicant 3-chloropropanediol (3-MCPD), which is detected in infant milk formulas at concentrations up to 1.0 mg/kg of fat extracted from the product.

The anisidine number correlates in a certain way with the accumulation of free aldehydes (hexenal, nonenal, 2,4-decadienal), which give the product foreign smells of fish, beans, etc.

The accumulation of thermostable secondary oxidation product mixture in the fat component is characteristic of the oxidation of fats during their heat treatment. The formation of highly polar compounds, insoluble in petroleum ether (CIPE), and epoxides were found in the study of deep-fried dough products as well as during the storage of confectionery products with a high-fat content—Kurabie cookies, shortbread cookies, Chak-chack, Creamy cake, and others. In a biological experiment on animals in our previous works, it was shown that fats containing more than 1% of CIPE with systematic consumption have a negative effect on the organs of the gastrointestinal tract, sharply reduce the level of erythrocytes and leukocytes in the blood, cause the accumulation of cholesterol and bilirubin [25]. The potential for such compounds to be formed in baby foods is a major concern.

Edible fats are an essential part of an infant's diet. Reproduction of the fatty acid composition of breast milk in the creation of infant formula is a complex scientific, technological and medical problem.

According to the requirements of Article 4 of TR CU 021/2011, adapted infant milk powder should be as close in chemical composition to human milk as possible in order to meet the physiological needs of infants for the necessary substances and energy. The fatty acid composition of breast milk is characterized by a relatively high content of polyunsaturated fatty acids (PUFA), the concentration of which in mature human milk is 12–15 times higher than in cow's milk (0.4–0.5 g/100 ml versus 0.009 g/100 ml). In the infant's body, unsaturated fatty acids are either synthesized to a limited extent (monounsaturated) or not synthesized at all (PUFA) while these compounds perform the most important plastic and metabolic functions. Of the greatest importance for young children are representatives of the ω-3 and ω-6 PUFA families, of which the most significant are α-linolenic and linoleic acids. In breast milk, the ratio of PUFAs of the ω-6 and ω-3 families is optimum and ranges from 10:1 to 7:1. Under the influence of the enzyme delta-6 desaturase, these compounds are converted into long-chain polyunsaturated fatty acids which play a leading role in the development of the central nervous system of infants, the visual analyzer, the immune system, and the regulation of metabolic processes and inflammatory reactions [26, 27]. Comparative characteristics of the average composition of the predominant fatty acids of adapted infant milk formulas and human milk are presented in **Table 1**.

The data presented in **Table 1** indicate the presence of gadoleic acid C20: 1 and a sufficiently high amount of linolenic acid C18: 3 in the "IN", "IM", "IL" mixtures, which might contain non-erucid rapeseed oil. According to the analysis of the fatty acid composition, the "IN", "IM", "IL" mixtures may have almost identical recipes.

From the data presented it can be seen that the mixtures were selected, first of all, according to the content of oleic and palmitic acids. "IX" sample contains 15–20% of coconut oil, "IS" sample contains 35% of coconut oil, the rest contain 30% of coconut oil. On the contrary, the "IS" mixture contains about 20% of palm oil, the "IX" sample contains 40–45% of palm oil, the rest contain 35–40% of palm oil.

The trivial name for a fatty acid, the number of carbon atoms in the chain, and the number of double bonds	Mass fraction of fatty acid in samples, %					
	Breast milk	IS	IN	IM	IL	IX
Caprylic C8: 0	0.17	3.2	2.2	2.2	2.0	0.9
Capric C10: 0	1.66	2.5	1.8	1.7	1.6	0.8
Lauric C12: 0	5.8	17.9	13.0	12.7	11.9	9.3
Myristic C14: 0	8.6	6.6	5.4	5.3	5.2	3.6
Palmitic C16: 0	21.0	8.4	18.9	18.6	19.2	24.4
Palmitoleic C16: 1	3.4	0.1	0.2	0.2	0.2	0.2
Stearic C18: 0	8.0	2.8	3.1	3.3	3.4	3.3
Oleic C18: 1	36.5	39.3	38.0	38.3	38.7	38.1
Linoleic acid C18: 2	10.8	16.9	14.1	14.1	14.2	16.2
Linolenic C18: 3	1.0	1.5	2.4	2.7	2.6	2.2
Arachidic C20: 0	0.21	0.2	0.3	0.3	0.3	0.3
Gadoleic C20: 1	0.20	0.2	0.4	0.4	0.4	0.40
Behenic C22: 0	0.10	0.4	0.2	0.2	0.3	0.2
Mass fraction of fat, %	4.4	3.6	3.4	3.3	3.3	3.6

Table 1.
Comparative characteristics of the average fatty acid composition of breast milk [11] and adapted milk powder.

The highest content of polyunsaturated acids (linoleic and linolenic) is in the "IS" and "IX" mixtures, while the most favorable ratio $\omega 6/\omega 3$ = 11: 1, corresponding to the characteristics of breast milk, was found in the "IS" mixture.

Mass fraction of the fat component ranges from 24.1% ("IM") to 27.7% ("IX").

Based on the research results, the fatty acid composition of adapted infant dry milk formulas by various manufacturers corresponds to the information indicated on the labels of the tested products.

Table 1 shows that the proposed mixtures contain an excessive amount of lauric acid and linoleic acid, with a relatively lower mass fraction of stearic acid. None of the studied samples in terms of the average composition of fatty acids fully corresponds to breast milk.

Infant formula was prepared for sensory analysis according to the recommendations indicated on the package, with a hydro module of one to three. Dispersion of dry mixtures in water occurred with the same intensity. The results of sensory analysis are presented in **Table 2**.

Baby food made from "IS", "IN", "IM", and "IL" mixtures had a fishy smell of varying intensity; "IX" mixture was more herbaceous, leguminous. The sweet taste was most explicit in the "IN" infant formula and least of all in the "IM" infant formula. The consistency of food systems varied slightly with colors ranging from white to cream.

Generally, it should be noted the unsatisfactory results of sensory analysis of varying degrees of food compositions intensity. The composition of the "IX"

Sample name	Taste	Odor	Consistency	Color
IS	Fishy aftertaste	Slightly fishy	Homogeneous, light, watery	Baked milk
IN	Sweet-salty with a fishy aftertaste	Poorly expressed fishy	Homogeneous, light, non-watery	Creamy white
IM	Slightly sweetish, creamy	Slight fishy smell	Homogeneous, light, non-watery	Creamy white
IL	Sweet and salty, with a metallic aftertaste	Slight fishy smell	Homogeneous, light, slightly watery	Creamy white
IX	Bean, with a cold synthetic flavor	Herbaceous	Homogeneous, light, non-watery	Light cream

Table 2.
The results of the sensory analysis of mixture samples.

Sample name	Acid number, mg KOH/g	Peroxidenumber, meq/kg	Anisidinenumber, cu	Mass fraction of oxidation products insoluble in petroleum ether, %	Mass fraction of oxidation products insoluble in petroleum ether, %
IS	0.5	0.4	1.9	0.3	25.6
IN	0.2	0.9	2.2	0.8	27.1
IM	0.6	1.4	3.6	1.0	31.1
IL	0.7	0.8	2.6	0.7	27.9
IX	0.4	1.1	2.9	0.6	26.3

Table 3.
Physicochemical indicators of the safety of adapted infant dry milk formulas.

mixture has the worst performance. Thus, a negative result of sensory analysis of the prepared infant formula indicates an unacceptable level of oxidation of the fat component and the need to change the shelf life of powdered infant formula. It has been proven that the weakening of antioxidant protection and uncontrolled enhancement of lipid oxidation is one of the important links in the pathogenesis of autonomic dysfunction, atopic dermatitis, dental pathology, diabetes mellitus, arthropathies, diseases of the gastrointestinal tract, urinary tract, etc. [28–30].

Physicochemical indicators of the safety of adapted infant dry milk formulas are presented in **Table 3**.

Analyzing the data in **Table 3** we can conclude that the safety indicator standardized by TR CU 033/2013 "On the safety of milk and dairy products" known as the peroxide number is within the normal range for all samples (no more than 4 meq/kg).

The limit value of the acid number for adapted milk powder is not determined by the legal requirements of the Customs Union. According to TR CU 024/2011 "For fat and oil products" for refined oils and their fractions, mixtures of refined oils, the acid number is normalized to no more than 0.6 mg KOH/g. For three of the five studied dry milk mixtures, the acid number does not exceed this indicator. In the "IM" and "IL" samples, the content of free fatty acids in the fat component is respectively 0.6 and 0.7 mg KOH/g.

The permissible value of the anisidine number (that shows the concentration of secondary oxidation products, i.e., aldehydes) is also not regulated by the legal requirements for adapted infant dry milk formulas. In GOST 1129-2013 "Sunflower oil." Specifications (as amended) this indicator is not more than 3 conventional units for Premium oils and Highest grade oils. In "IM" sample the anisidine number is 3.6 conventional units. The anisidine number shows the relative content of aldehydes. First of all, α- and β-unsaturated aldehydes which form yellow condensation products with reagents enter into the reaction with anisidine.

In addition, not only primary oxidation products are a risk factor but also oxidized fatty acids and their copolymerization products (CIPE), that is, secondary oxidation products. Therefore, in prototypes, this indicator was studied to identify a complete safety picture. The mass fraction of compounds insoluble in petroleum ether is regulated for waste frying fats according to SP 2.3.6.1079-01 at no more than 1%. This indicator has not yet been reflected when ensuring the safety of the fatty component of other food products, although there are a number of studies indicating the need for its regulation [31, 32]. In "IM" sample, immediately after opening, the mass fraction of CIPE was 1%. In biological studies on animals [33] it was noted that with the systematic consumption of fats containing more than 0.88% of CIPE, there are progressive negative pathological changes in the body (granular degeneration and hyperemia of the liver, desquamation processes in the intestinal wall, edema of the submucosal layer of the intestine, change in blood picture). Such changes indicate an increase in the number of eosinophils and compounds that are leukotoxins which commonly leads to disruptions in the work of the antioxidant defense systems of the body.

Some studies [34] have shown that it is the isomers of epoxyoleic acid that have the properties of leukotoxins. According to some researchers [35], the formation of an epoxy ring occurs through the reaction of a double bond in a fatty acid chain with a hydroperoxide formed in another adjacent fatty acid chain. This mechanism explains the presence of an epoxy ring at the site of the double bond, and the concomitant formation of a hydroxy function from hydroperoxide in the adjacent fatty acid chain. The formation of epoxides is accelerated by the thermal treatment of unsaturated fats which is used in spray drying of dry milk formulas.

Estimating the concentration of epoxides can be proposed as an operational method for monitoring the safety of the fat component of dry milk mixtures and other food products. In the studied infant dry milk formulas, the content of epoxides was 25–31 mmol/kg at the time of opening the can.

It should be noted that all the studied parameters of hydrolysis and oxidation of fats are at the safest level in the "IN" mixture; the indicators of the "IX" mixture are closer to the critical values.

The research results were processed by generally accepted statistical methods using the SPSS statistical program. For the statistical analysis, the Student's *t*-test was used.

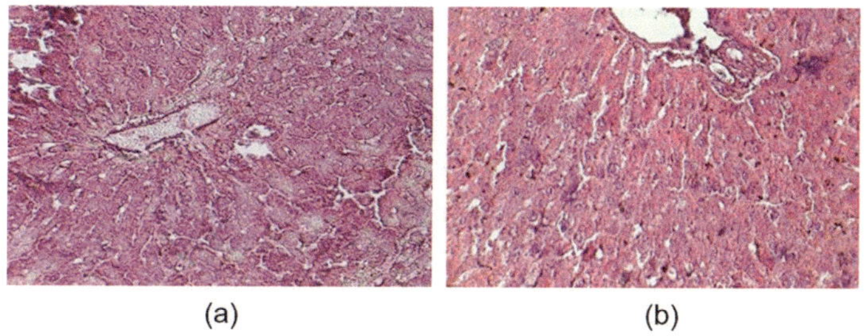

Figure 1.
Micrograph of the histological picture of the liver section of biomodels using "IN" sample (a) and the control group (b).

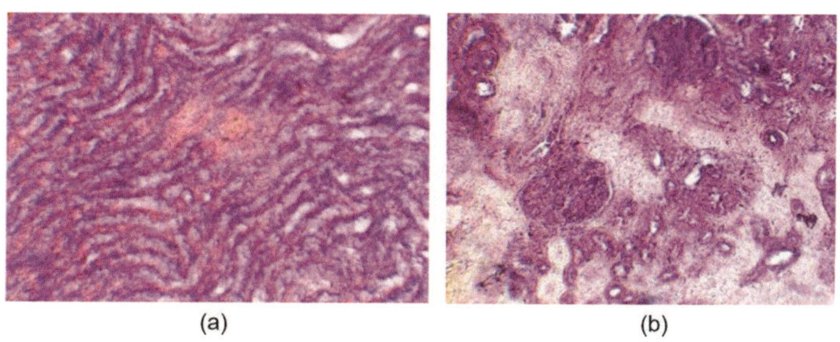

Figure 2.
Micrograph of the histological picture of a kidney picture of biomodels using "IS" (a) and "IM" (b) samples.

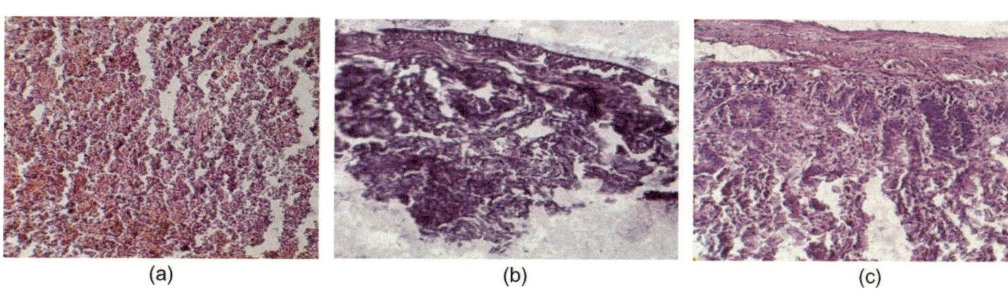

Figure 3.
Micrograph of a histological picture of a spleen section (a) and small intestine (b) of biomodels using "IL" sample, and of the large intestine of biomodels using "IX" sample (c).

In the future studies of the values of these indicators will be carried out at the end of the shelf-life period of the opened can.

3.1 Results of the second stage of research

The histological picture indicating changes occurring with a pronounced intensity is presented on micrographs (**Figures 1–3**). A detailed description of the histological picture of the tissues of the studied organs of the biomodels is presented in **Table 4**.

Structural disorders were most noticeable in Groups 4 and 5, while only in Group 1 the presence of intertubular hemorrhages was detected.

Severe suppression of lymphoid tissue in the spleen was detected in biomodels in Groups 4 and 5 and to a lesser extent in Group 1. Among all the cases studied, the structure of the wall of the small intestine was most disturbed primarily in Groups 4

Organ	Group 1IS	Group 2IN	Group 3IM	Group 4IL	Group 5IX	Control Group
Liver	Hyperemia, focal granular dystrophy, beam structure is moderately expressed.	Vessels are filled with blood, diffuse granular degeneration of hepatocytes, edema of Dissespaces, the beam structure is poorly visible.	Beam structure is poorly visible, diffuse hydropic dystrophy in combination with granular dystrophy, edematous phenomena in the tissues.	Beam structure is absent, granular degeneration of hepatocytes, hyperemia, edema of organ tissue.	Focal hydropic dystrophy in combination with granular degeneration of hepatocytes, the beam structure is poorly visible, hyperemia and tissue edema.	Beam structure is preserved, vessels are desolate, granular degeneration of hepatocytes.
Kidney	Focal hydropic dystrophy in combination with granular dystrophy. Granular dystrophy of the epithelium of the tubules, the accumulation of erythrocytes between them.	Focal hydropic dystrophy in combination with granular dystrophy of the tubular epithelium. Swellingofthevascularglomeruli.	Severe hydropic dystrophy in combination with granular dystrophy of the tubular epithelium, the vascular glomeruli are markedly enlarged.	Diffuse hydropic dystrophy in combination with granular dystrophy of the epithelium of the tubules, the vascular glomeruli are enlarged.	Focal hydropic dystrophy, a significant increase in vascular glomeruli with a decrease in the lumen of the Shumlyansky capsule.	Focal hydropic dystrophy in combination with granular dystrophy of the epithelium of the tubules, the vascular glomeruli are enlarged up to the complete disappearance of the lumen of the Shumlyansky capsule.
Spleen	Thinning of the lymphoid tissue of the follicles.	Perivascular edema, moderate loss of lymphocytes in the follicles.	Some rarefaction of the lymphoid tissue of the follicles.	Decrease in the number and size of follicles with thinning of the lymphoid tissue.	Follicles are not expressed, lymphoid tissue is poorly visible.	Moderate perivascular edema and loss of lymphocytes in the follicles.
Small intestine	Slight swelling of the organ wall.	Edema of the mucous membrane and deformation of the glands.	Edema of the organ wall and deformation of the glands.	Edema of the organ wall and deformation of the glands.	Moderate edema of the mucous membrane.	Edema of the organ wall and some deformation of the glands.

Organ	Group 1IS	Group 2IN	Group 3IM	Group 4IL	Group 5IX	Control Group
Colon	Edema of the mucous membrane.	Severe edema of the mucous membrane and deformation of the glands.	Edema of the mucous membrane and deformation of the glands.	Edema and deformation of the glands.	Edem and deformation of the glands.	Edema of the mucous membrane and fragmentation of some glands.

Table 4.
Histopathological changes in the internal organs of biomodels.

and 5 and, to a lesser extent, in Groups 2 and 3. The large intestine had pronounced disturbances in the structure of the wall in the form of edema and deformation of the glands in Groups 2 and 4.

4. Conclusion

Breast milk is the natural and most physiological nutrition for a child from the first days of their life. Its composition goes beyond simple nutritional support and is the most important postnatal factor in the metabolic and immunological programming of health. A high nutritional and functional potential of breast milk has been established indicating the biological advantage and fundamental indispensability of breastfeeding for the optimum development of both healthy and sick child. However, a significant proportion of women for various reasons are unable to provide their child with natural feeding. In these cases, it is important to use optimum, high-quality, and safe bottle-feeding. As a result of the study of fat component safety of the adapted infant dry milk formulas "IM", "IS", "IN", "IL", "IX" it was found that the qualitative composition of the fat fraction corresponds to that stated on the package. None of the samples under study in terms of the average composition of prevailing fatty acids fully corresponds to the composition of human milk. According to an important indicator, that is, the ratio of polyunsaturated fatty acids ω6/ω3, the "IS" mixture is distinguished by the optimum value (11:1).

As for the organoleptic characteristics food systems made from dry mixtures "IS", "IN", "IM", and "IL" had a fishy smell of varying intensity whereas "IX" mixture had a more herbaceous smell. Sweet taste was most pronounced in the "IN" formula and least of all in the "IM" formula. The consistency varied slightly, the color varied from white to cream. A negative organoleptic evaluation commonly indicates an unacceptable level of oxidation of the fat component of dry milk mixtures that causes the need to adjust the shelf life of dry milk mixtures.

Safety indicators of the fat component regulated by TR CU 021/2011, TR CU 024/2011, TR CU 033/2013 are not fully respect the safety requirements for the fat component of adapted dry milk mixtures since there are no standards for the most important safety indicators of fats, that is, the content of secondary oxidation products CIPE and epoxides. According to our opinion, the studies carried out necessitate further research of the parameters of the adapted dry milk mixtures fat component during storage after the package is opened by the consumer.

Histopathological changes were most regularly observed in the studied organs of Group 5 biomodels. Slightly less intensity of pathologies was expressed in Group 4. At the same time, in almost all other groups of biomodels, pathological processes of varying severity were detected in organs, although in some cases it is possible to assume their reversibility.

Thus, the conducted biological experiment previously proved that the use of "IX" and "IL" mixtures has a certain negative impact on the internal organs of biomodels.

The revealed information requires further study using modern research methods. The data obtained indicate the need for a precise evaluation of the production technology, packaging, and storage of adapted infant dry milk formulas, as well as the advisability of improving the legal regulation of the Russian Federation and the Customs Union, in order to strengthen and control the safety of adapted infant dry milk formulas, fat component, and changes in the shelf life of these products.

Author details

Ekaterina Yurievna Volf[1], Inna Vladimirovna Simakova[1*],
Andrey Anatolyevich Terentyev[2], Aleksandr Sergeevich Fedonnikov[3],
Nina Viktorovna Bolotova[3], Gloria Vladimirovna Guzeeva[4]
and Viktor Veniaminovich Zakrevsky[5]

1 Department of Food Technologies, Saratov State Agrarian University Named After N.I. Vavilov, Saratov, Russia

2 Department of Morphology, Pathology of Animals and Biology, Saratov State Agrarian University Named After N.I. Vavilov, Saratov, Russia

3 Saratov State Medical University Named After V.I. Razumovsky, Saratov, Russia

4 Pediatric Gastroenterology and Endoscopy of the Ministry of Health of the Saratov Region, Saratov Regional Children's Clinical Hospital, Saratov, Russia

5 Department of Food Hygiene, North-Western State Medical University Named After I.I. Mechnikov, St. Petersburg, Russia

*Address all correspondence to: simakovaiv@yandex.ru

References

[1] Gmoshinskaya MV, Surzhik AV, Ya KI, Georgieva OV, Safronova AI, Pustograev NN, et al. Indicators of physical and psychomotor development of infants in the first months of life who received an adapted milk mixture with prebiotics, nucleotides and long-chain polyunsaturated fatty acids [electronic resource], Abramova T.V. [and others]. Questions of Practical Pediatrics. 2015;(3):24-31

[2] Barabash NA, Melnikova UV, Pozhenko VV, Hypogalactia. Modern methods of correction and prevention: Guidelines. Tomsk: OOO "Offset Center". 2016:28

[3] Tutelyan VA, Kon IY, editors. Infant Food: A Guide for Doctors. 4th ed. Moscow, MIA: Rev. and add; 2017. p. 784

[4] Petrenko AV. Modern approaches to artificial feeding of children. In: Petrenko AV, editor. New Science: Experience, Traditions, Innovations: International Scientific Periodical Following the Results of the International Scientific and Practical Conference (August 12, 2016, Omsk)., Part 2. Sterlitamak: AMI; 2016. pp. 13-17

[5] Gould JF, Roberts RM, Makrides M. The influence of Omega-3 long-chain polyunsaturated fatty acid, docosahexaenoic acid, on child behavioral functioning: A review of randomized controlled trials of DHA supplementation in pregnancy, the neonatal period and infancy. Nutrients. 2021;**13**(2):415. DOI: 10.3390/nu13020415

[6] Koletzko B. Human milk lipids. Annals of Nutrition and Metabolism. 2016;**69**(Suppl 2):28-40. DOI: 10.1159/000452819. Epub 2017 Jan 20

[7] Verfuerden ML, Dib S, Jerrim J, Fewtrell M, Gilbert RE. Effect of long-chain polyunsaturated fatty acids in infant formula on long-term cognitive function in childhood: A systematic review and meta-analysis of randomised controlled trials. PLoS One. 2020;**15**(11):e0241800. DOI: 10.1371/journal.pone.0241800

[8] Verfürden ML, Gilbert R, Lucas A, Jerrim J, Fewtrell M. Effect of nutritionally modified infant formula on academic performance: Linkage of seven dormant randomised controlled trials to national education data. BMJ. 2021;**375**:e065805. DOI: 10.1136/bmj-2021-065805

[9] Shilina NM. An expert look at the role of fats in baby food. Pediatric Pharmacology. 2014;**11**(1):38-42

[10] Baby Nutrition. A Guide for Physicians Ed. V.a. Tutel'yana, I. Ya. Konya. 4th ed. Moscow: Medical Information Agency LLC; 2017. p. 784

[11] Martin CR, Ling PR, Blackburn GL. Review of infant feeding: Key features of breast milk and infant formula. Nutrients. 2016;**8**(5):279. Published 2016, May 11. DOI: 10.3390/nu8050279

[12] Phipps R, Lynch B, Stannard DR, Gilby B, Baldwin N, Mikš MH, et al. Genotoxicity and neonatal subchronic toxicity assessment of a novel mixture of the human-identical milk oligosaccharides lacto-N-fucopentaose I and 2′-fucosyllactose. Journal of Applied Toxicology. 2020;**41**(4):632-649. DOI: 10.1002/jat.4071

[13] Rodríguez-Alcalá LM, Calvo MV, Fontecha J, Alonso L. Alterations in the fatty acid composition in infant formulas and ω3-PUFA enriched UHT Milk during storage. Food. 2019;**8**:163

[14] Timby N, Domellöf M, Lönnerdal B, Hernell O. Comment on "safety and tolerance evaluation of Milk fat globule membrane-enriched infant formulas: A randomized controlled multicenter non-inferiority trial in healthy term infants". Clinical Medical Insights Pediatrics. 2015 Jun;**18**(9):63-64. DOI: 10.4137/CMPed.S27185

[15] MacMahon S, Begley TH, Diachenko GW. Occurrence of 3-MCPD and glycidyl esters in edible oils in the United States. Food Additives & Contaminants, Part A: Chemistry, Analysis, Control, Exposure & Risk Assessment. 2013;**30**:2081-2092

[16] Kent G. Regulating fatty acids in infant formula: Critical assessment of U.S. policies and practices. International Breastfeeding Journal. 2014;**9**(1):2. DOI: 10.1186/1746-4358-9-2

[17] Makarenko MA, Malinkin AD, Bokov DO, Bessonov VV. Monochloropropanediols, glycidol and their esters in children's nutrition. Vopr.det. dietol. (Pediatric Nutrition). 2019;**17**(1):38-48. (In Russian)

[18] ISO 18363-1:2015 Animal and vegetable fats and oils. Determination of Fatty-Acid-Bound Chloropropanediols (MCPDs) and Glycidol by GC/MS —Method Using Fast Alkaline Transesterification and Measurement for 3-MCPD and Differential Measurement for Glycidol2015. DOI: 10.20953/1727-5784-2019-1-38-48

[19] Leigh J, MacMahon S. Occurrence of 3- monochloropropanediol esters and glycidyl esters in commercial infant formulas in the United States. Food Addit Contam: Part A. 2017;**34**(3):356-370

[20] Becalski A, Feng S, Lau BP-Y, Zhao T. A pilot survey of 2- and 3-monochloropropanediol and glycidol fatty acid esters in foods on the Canadian market 2011 -2013. Food Composition and Analysis. 2015;**37**:58-66

[21] Wang W, Yang J, Qi W, Yang H, Wang C, Tan B, et al. Lipidomic profiling of high-fat diet-induced obesity in mice: Importance of cytochrome P450-derived fatty acid epoxides. Obesity (Silver Spring). 2017;**25**:132-140

[22] Li P, Oh da Y, Bandyopadhyay G, et al. LTB4 promotes insulin resistance in obese mice by acting on macrophages, hepatocytes and myocytes. Nature Medicine. 2015;**21**:239-247

[23] Lilly R. Pathohistological Technique and Practical Histology., Eng-Rus Translation; ed. and with a Foreword by AM of AMN, V.V. Portugalova., Moscow : Mir. 1969. p. 512

[24] Merkulov, Grigory Andreevich. Course of pathological and histological techniques [Text]. - 5th ed., Rev. and additional - Leningrad: Medicine. Leningrad. department, 1969. - 423 p. : ill.; 22 cm

[25] Simakova IV. Scientific and Applied Aspects of Safety Fast Food: Thesis. Orel: Doctor of Technical Sciences; 2015. p. 338

[26] Zakharova YA, Dmitrieva IN, Gordeeva EA. Membrane of fat globules of milk: Innovative discoveries already today. Russian Bulletin of Perinatology and Pediatrics. 2015;(6):15-21

[27] Janssen CI, Kiliaan AJ. Long-chain polyunsaturated fatty acids (LCPUFA) from genesis to senescence: The influence of LCPUFA on neural development, aging, and neurodegeneration. Progress in Lipid Research. 2014;**53**:1-17. DOI: 10.1016/j.plipres.2013.10.002. Epub 2013 Oct 24

[28] Ozcagli E, Alpertunga B, Fenga C, Berktas M, Tsitsimpikou C, Wilks MF,

et al. Effects of 3-monochloropropane-1,2-diol (3-MCPD) and its metabolites on DNA damage and repair under in vitro conditions. Food and Chemical Toxicology. 2016;**89**:1-7

[29] Kazimirko VK, Maltsev VI. The Antioxidant System and its Functioning in the Human Body. Electronic resource., Access: http://www.health-ua.com/; 2004 Date of access: February 28, 2019

[30] Kurashvili, V.A. Relief of oxidative stress using natural antioxidants, electronic resource. Access: http://vitadoctor.com.ua. Date of access: February 28, 2019

[31] Simakova IV, Perkel RL, Zakrevkiy VV, Kutkina MN. Investigation of the intensity of pathogenesis depending on the oxidation state of palm oil. Nutrition Issues. 2016;**85**(2):36

[32] Simakova IV, Eliseev YY, Perkel RL, Domnitsky IY, Terentyev AA, Strizhevskaya VN, et al. Assessment of the sanitary and technological safety of the fatty component of some types of snacks and flour confectionery products with a long shelf life. Saratov Journal of Medical Scientific Research. 2016;**12**(3):333-339

[33] Simakova IV. Scientific and Applied Aspects of Ensuring the Safety of Fast Food Products, Thesis for a Doctor's of Eechnical Sciences Degree. Orel: Federal State Budgetary Educational Institution of Higher Education Prioksky State University; 2015. p. 462

[34] Goicoechea E, Guillen MD. Analysis of hydroperoxydes, aldehydes and epoxydes by ^{1}H nuclear magnetic resonance in sunflower oil oxidized at 70 and 100°C. Agricultural Journal of Food Chemistry. 2010;**58**:6234-6245

[35] Grüneis V, Fruehwirth S, Zehl M, Ortner J, Schamann A, König J, et al. Simultaneous analysis of Epoxidized and Hydroperoxidized Triacylglycerols in canola oil and margarine by LC-MS. Journal of Agricultural and Food Chemistry. 2019;**67**(36):10174-10184. DOI: 10.1021/acs.jafc.9b03601. Epub 2019 Aug 28